TRIGGER™
The mental health & wellbeing publisher

T0145628

THE AUTHOR

Hope Virgo suffered with anorexia for four years before being admitted to hospital in 2007. She was hospitalised for a year, and since being discharged has fought to stay well. Hope now lives and works in London and has a keen interest in fitness and maintaining good mental health. She enjoys running marathons and now has a much healthier perception of food. It means that after years of fixating on the calorific content of everything, Hope can relax and enjoy what she eats. She is standing tall and looking to the future with confidence.

First published in 2017
This edition published in 2023 by Trigger Publishing
An imprint of Shaw Callaghan Ltd

UK Office
The Stanley Building
7 Pancras Square
Kings Cross
London N1C 4AG

US Office
On Point Executive Center, Inc
3030 N Rocky Point Drive W
Suite 150
Tampa, FL 33607
www.triggerhub.org

A CIP catalogue record for this book is available upon request from the British
Library
ISBN: 9781837963690
Ebook ISBN: 9781837963706

Cover design and typeset by Fusion Graphic Design Ltd
Cover Image by Vicki Sharp Photography

Trigger Publishing encourages diversity and different viewpoints. However, all
views, thoughts and opinions expressed in this book are the author's own and are
not necessarily representative of us as an organization.

All material in this book is set out in good faith for general guidance and no liability
can be accepted for loss or expense incurred in following the information given. In
particular this book is not intended to replace expert medical or psychiatric advice.
It is intended for informational purposes only and for your own personal use and
guidance. It is not intended to act as a substitute for professional medical advice.
The author is not a medical practitioner nor a counsellor, and professional advice
should be sought if desired before embarking on any health-related programme.

Dedicated to all those who are suffering, all those supporting sufferers and those who just need to start believing in themselves that they are worth the fight. Keep fighting.

INTRODUCTION

HITTING ROCK BOTTOM

'Do you ever get the feeling that you're in deep and sinking?
That you're in way over your head and out of your depth?
Screams bleating, you teeter, topple, flop, crippled with doubt,
and there ain't no way in hell you'll ever figure this out.'

I stood in the hospital doorway, my hair thinning, my skin a yellowish colour. I was wearing a short denim skirt and a pink jumper that drowned me. Tears were welling in my eyes as Mum signed me in. I begged her to let me come home. I just wanted one more chance.

I promised I would begin to eat. But Mum couldn't take any more of my lies. I hated her then, and everyone around me. I couldn't understand why they were interfering in my life. Yes, I had lost a bit of weight, but I wasn't that skinny. I was nowhere near thin enough to die ...

The last week flashed before my eyes. My heart had nearly stopped. An emergency ECG showed that it was losing muscle fast. And still my weight kept on dropping. If I didn't start to eat soon, I would die. It was that simple.

We sat in one of the family rooms at the Riverside Unit in Bristol and talked about my history. My parents bickered. Nothing anyone said seemed to matter. Then I was taken next door and weighed. I wondered if the scales would be accurate? Would they show how good at anorexia I was? Did it mean I was a successful anorexic now that I was being told my heart was about to fail?

For the first time in years, my anger drained away and I was afraid.

Just forty-eight hours earlier, I'd been at school with my friends. How had it come to this? I thought back over the months of working out in my bedroom at all hours, or sneaking off to the gym before school. All the hours of 'showering' after dinner when really, I was throwing up; the sound of the shower drowning out the guttural noise of my forced vomiting. I had been getting good at keeping my anorexia secret. But now, just as I was getting into the swing of it, I was admitted to a mental health hospital.

Had I really lost all control. Had I hit rock bottom?

Was I really about to die?

PART 1

STANDING TALL

CHAPTER 1

BACK WHERE IT ALL BEGAN

Jennifer Hope Virgo died of heart failure, as a result of anorexia nervosa, aged seventeen.

That's what my death certificate would have read, had things ended differently.

Was I born with a genetic susceptibility to anorexia, or did life make me anorexic?

My story began on 8 May 1990 in St Michael's Hospital in Bristol. I was the middle child of five. Kate and James are older than me; Samuel and Mollie are younger. Growing up, I felt so lucky to have so many brothers and sisters to play with, and I loved our house and garden. We'd spend hours running around, playing ball games, and climbing the trees in the summer. Whenever we lost our ball over the fence, we'd take it in turns to dash across the grounds of the residential home next door, daring each other to see how far we could go without getting caught! It felt like a little act of rebellion, but then I was already getting a reputation for being a rebellious child ...

When I was four, I had amazing long hair, like a mermaid. Kate loved it. We'd sit on her bed and she would brush it for hours. It always felt so nice, and I enjoyed spending time with my big sister, so I can't quite explain what I did next. For some bizarre reason I ran off and hid, and then, quite calmly, I took some scissors and started cutting great chunks out of my hair. I was caught while scalping myself, but it was too late; I'd managed to hack off half my hair. My sister was devastated. But at the time, I didn't care at all. I felt absolutely no emotion until I went back to school. There was a girl there who had such long hair she could sit on it, and the moment I saw her it hit me: I was absolutely gutted mine had gone, and I'd been left with a short bob. I wanted my long hair back so badly!

As my birthday was in the spring, I would often have swimming pool parties. But I'd just sit on the edge of the pool and dangle my feet. It wasn't that I didn't like swimming; I just hated being in a swimsuit. I can't ever remember not feeling self-conscious about it. Mum bought me a "tankini" so that I didn't feel quite so exposed, but it didn't make me feel any better. I used to look longingly at the other girls around me, wishing I looked more like them. I was desperate to be their shape.

And if there were others who were different sizes, I would wonder why they weren't all feeling as self-conscious as I was. If I absolutely had to go swimming, I'd wear shorts and a t-shirt over my costume. By secondary school, I'd get out of swimming by saying I was on my period, or I'd forgotten my stuff. I'd rather face an hour of detention than risk being seen in a swimming costume.

I much preferred cycling. The day before Mollie was born, we cycled to Bath. Cycling was the one and only thing we used to enjoy doing as a family. We'd stop for ice creams along the way and enjoy a pub lunch. Getting out on our bikes was always such a wonderful relief from home life. It meant that we would be able to have our own space and time apart while still doing the "family thing". We all really relaxed when we did these types of activities and it was so refreshing just cycling along, pretending to have no care in the world. So even though Mum was very pregnant – and Mollie was already overdue – she didn't want to miss out. I remember the thrill of racing each other along the way. We laughed a lot and enjoyed the feeling of being part of a close-knit family. But that feeling of closeness never lasted very long. By the evenings we would be home and having heated family discussions, each of us taking the role to wind up someone else.

That night I slept on a mattress in Mum's room. I often slept in there because I had such vivid dreams that left me feeling scared and alone in the middle of the night.

When I woke at about 6.30 am, I saw that Mum's bed was empty. Mum and Dad rarely slept in the same room any more, so I checked Dad's room. He was gone too, but our neighbour had arrived to look after us. It could only mean one thing ... Mollie was on her way!

Part of me was so excited to welcome Mollie home. It was hard for the first few weeks as we had endless visitors, but we all loved her instantly. I hoped her arrival would bring Mum and Dad closer together, but deep down, I already knew their marriage was falling apart. I was becoming more aware of the arguments, which had become a routine part of our family life.

I guess I learnt to switch off from the bickering. In a way, I became completely unengaged with any sort of emotion. It just seemed easier that way. I didn't need to get involved; I could just push all my feelings, my worries, and my sadness straight under a mat. I liked it that way.

I was fantastic at showing people I was okay and pretending to be whatever they wanted me to be. Wearing this metaphorical mask from such an early age was hard work, but it guarded me from pain and made my life so much easier to manage. I would watch on as my family argued, occasionally joining in. But most of the time I would take their constant bickering as an opportunity to think about other things in life.

I know it was tough for Mum. She would look at me with love in her eyes and see a blank face staring back at her. It looked as if I didn't reciprocate her love. As if, at age nine, my emotions were already broken.

The answer? Therapy. What else?! Little did I know that this was just the start of a young life full of talking to therapists, counsellors and doctors.

Every week, Mum would take me to see a therapist. I would go every Thursday lunchtime. The therapist was a little bit of a hippy and I didn't really warm to her. I didn't understand why I was there or what she was trying to make me do. I had to paint lots of pictures for her, and I hated it because I was so unartistic! She'd ask me to write my worries and bad habits on little pieces of paper and put them in a tissue box. It was supposed to help me feel free of them. But it didn't work. I definitely wasn't brave enough to access my deeper feelings like that. So instead, I thought, *What worries and habits would other people come up with? What is the right and wrong and answer? What would all my friends do in this situation?*

I was already a very matter-of-fact person, and when my emotions got too much for me I boxed them up, masked my feelings and just got on with things. And after six months of the therapy, nothing had changed for me in the slightest. I liked how I lived my life and I didn't think it was a bad thing.

I went to the same junior school as Kate, but I wasn't as academic as her, so I spent most of my childhood feeling inferior to her. Teachers would compare us, or announce to the classroom that 'Kate wouldn't have done it like that'. And so I was delighted when my parents moved me to a different secondary school, where I settled in quickly. I made new friends and did all the things "normal" girls do.

But my rebellious streak didn't go away. I used to get into trouble for talking too much, or rolling my eyes at the teachers. I thought a lot of lessons were a complete waste of time, and I didn't keep my thoughts to myself. It might not have been the most sensible thing to vocalise them so openly, but I didn't care.

I worked hard anyway. I couldn't help it; we were a hard-working family. Dad worked long hours as a lawyer and the rest of us had to get up to do music practice for an hour every day before school. The enjoyment of music didn't come easily to me; practising was boring, and exams just felt like another tick-box exercise. My biggest escape was sport. James had always been sporty, and I liked that we were both good at it. My main sport was netball, but team sports frustrated me. I used to get overly competitive and frustrated with teammates who didn't work hard enough.

As life got harder, I started to crave physical activity more and more. It was my relief from all the pain I was feeling inside.

Maybe that's why I decided to join the cross-country team. I loved everything about running; I especially liked proving myself against other runners. I never really thought I was obsessed with it, but I suppose the signs were there. I liked to work hard and I was driven and determined – but what athletes weren't? I was certainly committed to training and dreamt of being a professional athlete, so when I look back at all my issues around food, it's hard not to feel frustrated that I missed out on opportunities to pursue my dream. But it wasn't to be. Within a few years, my life was falling apart ...

CHAPTER 2

LIVING A LIFE DOMINATED BY FOOD

By the age of twelve, I was already self-conscious about my weight. I wasn't as thin as the other girls at school. My parents kept saying I would thin out as I got taller, but I didn't think that was going to happen. Shortly after my thirteenth birthday I got sick. I didn't eat properly for a few weeks and lost a fair bit of weight. It was fab! I was finally thinning out and people around me were saying how much better I looked for it. Some might say this is where my insecurities began and I developed my driven personality. But at that point in my life, I still felt in control of my eating.

After people noticed my weight loss, I started to feel better about myself, and began to think more about what I was eating. A few girls skipped their school lunch, and I joined them a few times, saying I didn't feel hungry. We'd lie to the teachers when they asked us if we had eaten, or hide in the toilets until the coast was clear.

It was easy to miss meals, and it was a quick way to force my calorie intake down. When I did go for lunch, I'd give half of it away to anyone who wanted it. There was a points system and you had ten points to spend. A bread roll would be one, a main meal five, sweets three, and an apple three. Most people would try to max out the amount of food per point, but I spent my time seeing how little I could get. When I did end up getting too much, I would pick my way through it, drop it on the floor, or give it away. No one suspected a thing. And I definitely began to feel better about myself.

It was easy to find new diet tips on Google, and I quickly became an expert. The frustrating thing for me now is that I learnt too well! I know the calories of pretty much everything. If I have a bad day, I can't help but add up all the calories on my plate. Great for pub quiz questions perhaps, but a real burden to bear if you're fighting anorexia.

My thoughts gradually became dominated by food. I would spend hours cooking in the kitchen without ever eating any of it. Mum would get angry about all the food I was wasting, but I wondered if she was secretly envious of my self-restraint.

I don't know why I had the constant urge to cook, as I knew while I was doing it that I wasn't going to eat it. Perhaps it was because I could fiddle with it without having the pressure of eating it. Another part of me longed for the food. I hated food, yet I thought about it all the time. It was easier to think about food than to think about what was actually going on in life. I would cook for hours – cakes, cookies, whatever took my fancy. As I did it, I got this sense of satisfaction from not eating the food afterwards. I suddenly had control: I could bake a cake and not touch even a crumb of it.

Things were getting harder at home, arguments were becoming more and more frequent. There was always so much tension and I found it really hard. James was angry a lot of the time and I think he struggled a lot with his emotions too. He would walk around the house in the mornings with his headphones in, just ignoring everything. He argued a lot with Mum and Dad; they'd wind each other up and then someone would suddenly snap. There was always so much drama at home. It became part of normal life, but deep down I hated it. I hated feeling so unsure of what each day would bring, what arguments there would be and what was going on for everyone. One evening, he punched a wall – shattering all the bones in his hand – and then he stormed out of the house.

'We have to go and find him,' I told Dad hours later, when he still hadn't come home. As we drove around the neighbourhood, I looked into the houses, watching the residents as we sped by. I wondered what was happening in their lives and what was going on in their minds. It struck me then that we never really know anyone. I felt lost and alone, as if nobody really understood or cared for me. Perhaps I didn't even want them to care.

When we finally found James, we took him straight to A&E. Dad was lost for words. I was hurting inside, and as I looked in to James' eyes, I saw a lost, young boy, alone and afraid of his own strength. I saw it is my job to try and fix this family dynamic and try and make it all okay for James and everyone else at home. I didn't mind spending time walking with him late in to the night, trying to keep the peace and calm everyone down.

Mum and Dad's relationship was splintering. I remember spending evenings sitting on the stairs while they argued, or hiding away in Mollie's room, trying to stop her listening. Sometimes the arguments would escalate to the point where Mum would pack a bag, grab things for Mollie, and say she was leaving. Then Dad would break down and ask her to stay.

Dad wasn't like me. While I kept my emotions locked up, he wore his heart on his sleeve. I'd even see him well up at sad films. Being so in touch with his emotions wasn't such a bad thing, but Mum was very different. She certainly wore the trousers in their relationship, and I really looked up to her. She was career driven and determined. When she had ideas, she made them happen. I often wondered if that made my dad feel threatened.

It frustrated me how much Mum and Dad argued, but it frustrated me more that nothing was ever resolved. Everyone would go to bed with the nasty words still running through their heads. Next morning, we'd all have to go about our business as if nothing had happened. And again, I'd feel like I had to fix everything and make more effort at breakfast to keep the peace.

17

I took on the worries of the world and spent hours trying to resolve them. It was my responsibility in a way; I had to be there for my brothers and sisters. It was a huge responsibility, but right from an early age, I accepted it. It was what I did.

Around that time, I met someone.

At first, he seemed lovely. He was an older man who worked at the church. His name was Steven and he was quite a bit older than me. Looking back, I can see that it was a twisted, abusive relationship. But at the time it felt almost normal. Or maybe I was just too cut off from my feelings to care?

In the time we were together, I hardly existed as a thinking individual. I didn't assert myself with him. I just did everything I could to please him. I got used to being hurt and shouted at.

He made me do things sexually that I didn't want to do. And afterwards, he'd blame me for everything. 'It's all your fault!' he'd shout at me. It was my fault he'd touched me where I didn't want to be touched. And then, after the shouting, he'd break down in tears and apologise. He'd beg my forgiveness and promise me it'd never, ever happen again. But it always did. We were together for eight months before I summoned up the courage to end it. This was so hard to do; I was terrified of what would follow.

The images haunted me then. And even now, when the memories resurface, I wake in the night, feeling dead inside.

It affected me in other ways too. The cycle of abuse and the ongoing erosion of my feelings left me unable to assert myself in difficult situations. I wish I'd been able to stand up for myself, but I didn't have the courage to do it.

After I went into hospital, Mum tried to prosecute – she kept calling it sexual abuse. Other people suggested it would be difficult to act on my allegations unless I was willing to pursue a criminal case. But I knew that I just didn't have the energy to do that, so I left it. I guess back then I didn't know the knock-on effect it would have on my life.

When I was fifteen, I volunteered at a kids' club and ended up running a girls' support group, focusing on developing self-esteem in girls from a deprived part of Bristol. I liked being able to help and the girls really looked up to me. Lots of them even wanted to be like me. I would spend hours talking things through with them and we'd cook healthy meals together. As soon as they went home, I'd worry about them until I saw them again the next week.

I just wanted my girls to learn to feel self-worth, to feel special. I loved being there, but deep down, I knew I was a fake – I preached one thing and practised something completely different. Even though I was a failure, I thought that I could still fix them. So that's what I did. I stopped caring about myself and spent my time supporting everyone else.

As I got older I spent more time away from my family, and when I was at home, I'd shut myself in my bedroom. I was content with my own company and hated people stepping foot inside my room. My friend Charlotte and I had recently painted it dark-green and cream. Half the room looked amazing, but we'd got bored halfway through, so the other half was a bit messy. My bed was a mattress on the floor, and I kept my diary hidden underneath it – hidden away from prying eyes.

Or so I thought.

I spent time every evening writing in my diary – everything from boy crushes, to arguments, to food tips and yearly goals (which always consisted of losing weight).

There was a bookcase jutting out from the wall so that the bed was hidden from the doorway. It gave me a feeling of privacy – this was my space and mine alone. My room wasn't anything special, but it was my sanctuary. I had all my belongings laid out, and I'd spend hours organising and re-organising them so they were all really neat.

One New Year's Eve, I spilt black nail varnish on my new carpet. I was so scared of Mum getting cross, so in desperation, I got Kate to help me scrub it with bleach. And then Dad came in and tried to help, but the damage had already been done. After that, my no-admittance policy went back into effect!

The family arguments continued, but they had started to feel like a part of everyday life. I don't know if it was a good thing or a bad thing, but I actually got used to them. I was numb to the sounds and the feelings of unhappiness, and I could tell which arguments would blow over and which ones would get worse as the night progressed. I got to the point where I almost didn't care what happened or what was said – as long as I wasn't involved.

And that's how I learnt to live my life. When people got too close or my emotions got too much for me, I learnt to box it all up and push people away. I switched off from all the unpleasant emotions and pretended to be fine. I was starting to find that exercising complete control over my food helped me manage my emotions too. More and more I was relying on my patented Hope Virgo defence mechanisms!

Even now, I get nervous about people knowing me and my feelings, and I prefer to steer conversations away from my emotions and focus on other people instead. Sometimes I'll just tell silly stories. As my friends and family will tell you, I remember all the minor details of other people's lives. And I just want to help. From volunteering in Thailand and at the Calais Refugee Camp, to checking in on people at work, supporting others makes me feel truly complete.

I probably came across as being emotionally mature, but in truth, I couldn't stand feeling my own emotions. I literally hated feeling anything. And that's when my anorexia came to the rescue … She taught me how to be numb from pain and hurt. She told me there was no point in spending time with people or getting to know them. Sooner or later, she said, they'd always hurt me. But she wouldn't ever let me down. She was there to build my confidence and protect me from a world of pain.

As my family life got harder, and as Mum and Dad's marriage strained to breaking point, I took on even more responsibility for my family. It didn't matter how tough the family arguments were, it didn't matter how scared I felt. I didn't want to show any sign of weakness. I didn't want people to know that I cared. And as the arguments raged, my mind wandered to food or exercise, and I spent hours Googling how to lose weight. It helped to distract me from reality and I preferred to spend mealtimes adding up the calories on my plate instead of taking part in the conversations. It helped me box up the family worries and arguments. I was starting to find that I would rather be on my own than embrace the reality of the world.

My anorexia gave me a kind of self-worth. I was so bad at life. I was so bad at saving my family. But I was going to be good at dieting and exercise. I was going to know everything that I needed to know about nutrition. And all that time researching gave me so much satisfaction.

I craved that sense of achievement. I wanted to switch off from my feelings, and my anorexia was helping me more and more. Over the weeks, months and years, my feelings of detachment became part of my identity. My control around food gave me direction and a new purpose. These new thoughts were merging and transforming into something more. They formed and became a new friend for me. A close friend. In fact, my best friend. She wasn't going to let me down or leave me like others did; instead she was going to help me conquer life.

She was just for me, my anorexia.

And this is her story as much as mine.

CHAPTER 3

WHY DIDN'T WE SPOT HOPE'S ANOREXIA?

by Caroline Virgo (Hope's mum)

In the 1990s there was so much less awareness of anorexia. It wasn't the accepted topic of discussion it is today. None of us really understood just how serious it was, and that's how Hope got more and more ill without us ever really knowing.

Hope was such an eagerly anticipated addition to our family. She spent the first few weeks of her life lying on my chest. Her body temperature had dropped quickly after birth, so I had to keep her warm. It was essential bonding time, of course, and I felt like I could already sense her personality starting to develop, even then. She seemed so alert and ready for life. In a hurry to get on with living, perhaps. She seemed so interested in life going on around her.

We were a tight-knit group in Hope's early years. Our family was growing, and we were happy. Yes, there were family disagreements, but there was a lot of love too. I can certainly remember some friction between Hope and James, but that was hardly surprising, given their contrasting personalities. Mealtimes in those early years were definitely more peaceful when they sat apart!

I am a good cook and I loved to present my family with home-cooked meals. We were already aware of the need to eat healthily (although in the 1990s there was quite a different view of what healthy food was). I wasn't unduly rigid about snacks between meals, and fruit was always available, so the children ate well and ate plenty.

Or so I thought ...

How could I have not noticed Hope skipping meals?

Breakfast time: with five children and a husband all heading off to work and school, I'd be in the kitchen from 6.45 am, making sure everyone got what they wanted. For the boys I'd make a cooked breakfast, and for the girls there'd always be plenty of cereal or toast. In amongst all the noise and rushing around, it would have been easy for Hope to slip under the radar.

School lunches: when your daughter goes to school with a lunch in her bag and comes home with an empty bag, you just assume they're eating everything. Why would you think otherwise?

Hope announced she was a vegetarian in her teens. Looking back, I know it was a tactic to avoid eating dinner, but she knew I would always have cooked whatever she wanted. She could have eaten "something" and vegetables, but by the summer of 2005 she was mostly eating salad.

Hope was a rebellious child. I don't think she'd deny that, or mind me saying it! She was certainly single-minded, with a tendency to do exactly what she wanted. My attempts to rein her in weren't always successful. Does it sound like I was an absent parent? I really wasn't. I certainly liked to please the people I loved – and I suppose I thought Hope was the same. So I trusted that she told me the truth about whatever she said she was doing.

I certainly wasn't happy about the "boy". Hope was quickly growing into a beautiful young woman and wanted to attract attention to herself. Inevitably, the attention she got was increasingly from boys.

Looking back, I shouldn't have let her be involved with Steven. I was lulled into a false sense of security by his friendly personality and his anxiousness to please. He was always so polite, and so interested in our family. But now I know that allowing her to see him was a huge mistake.

CHAPTER 4

LOSING CONTROL

I was thirteen years old when I first met Anorexia properly. And from that moment on, I was hers. She knew just how to make me feel better every time. And she was always there for me to talk to. She gave me this value and sense of purpose that I wasn't getting from anyone else and I thrived off everything she gave me. She was all I needed and wanted.

She motivated me each morning, and held me tight when I lay in bed, listening to my family arguing. I knew she'd never, ever let go.

After a few months of being friends, she encouraged me to skip a meal for the first time. It felt strange – a little bit rebellious even, but boy, the sense of achievement I got was immense. Imagine scoring the winning goal for your country, or winning gold medal after gold medal at the Olympics. That is how I felt. That's how she made me feel.

Before Anorexia, I had never really felt good enough for anyone. I never felt as if I could make people happy with my behaviour, or my grades at school. But I knew just how to please her.

'Just think,' she would say to me, 'if you felt that good when you skipped one meal, imagine how good you'd feel – how good *we'd* feel – if you skipped more.'

She was right. It did feel amazing. Empowering, almost. How could I resist her after that? She always knew just what to say.

Surviving off just one meal a day felt amazing. But that wasn't enough for us.

Surviving off a couple of pieces of toast felt incredible, and the feeling of satisfaction I had when I got to the end of the day and had eaten nothing was like nothing else.

It was so easy to do it at home. I would take ages getting ready for school, and lie to Mum that I'd already eaten something. Or I'd pour my cereal back into the box or just give it to the dog.

Then, in the evenings, I'd play sport after school, get home late and say I was too busy with my homework to eat. And if I had to have dinner? I'd just make sure my plate was full of vegetables so it looked like I had a huge portion, but really, it was all water-heavy, calorie-light nutrition.

It was all so easy. And the easier it got, the more I tried to miss meals. I was getting sneakier too. I lied about every single meal. Then every evening, I would record what I had eaten that day. After a few months, I bought a calorie book so I could track everything precisely. I spent time learning the ins and outs of calorific content. I wanted to know it all.

I was excited by my new friend, and I felt such a thrill every time she talked to me. She understood me and I understood her. She congratulated me whenever I did well, and I needed that validation.

Do you know how it feels to be so down on yourself? To have no concept of self-worth?

That's how I felt. Every day of my life. And then suddenly, Anorexia was there, making me feel valued. Making me feel like maybe, just maybe, I was good enough. It was a life-changing feeling.

I was content when I was with her. She distracted me from the world around me and the ongoing reality of an unhappy family. I would lie in bed in the evenings, listening to my parents arguing downstairs. And as soon as I felt anything, I would think about food, calories, exercise; listening to Anorexia kept me away from life. But I couldn't take this new relationship for granted. I knew I'd need to go on proving my worth if I wanted her to keep believing in me.

On Sunday nights, I'd go to choir practice and lie about eating there. Then I'd get home and wouldn't have anything to eat after church. Dad thought he was on to me, but the one time he picked me up on it, I shouted at him. I said I didn't want anything, and headed straight to bed. Yes, I felt bad for upsetting him, but I rationalised it by telling myself it was his fault for interfering. I didn't like conflict, but as I didn't know how to manage my emotions, my frustration came out in explosive ways if I felt like people were interfering.

One lunchtime I wanted to show her just how committed I was to losing weight. As a vast roast dinner was served up in front of me, with endless oil over the roast potatoes and calorific meat and gravy – I announced to the table that I was, in fact, a vegetarian, and I wouldn't be eating any of it. My family probably assumed it was just a phase, something that would pass within a week or two. Little did they know that this was the new me.

It's not easy to force a determined teenager to eat. So if anyone ever questioned my eating after that, I would make up reasons why I didn't want to eat, or couldn't eat. By the time I was fifteen, arguments at mealtimes had become the norm and I would often storm off from the table without a care in the world. They said I was being selfish for not eating. But I didn't care anymore. I was winning. We were winning. And I was showing my best friend that I was good at this. I wanted to make her happy. That was all that mattered.

Looking back, it makes me feel a little bit guilty, even a bit sad. I know what a nightmare I was to live with. But at the time, I was a self-centred girl, preoccupied by my obsession with food, willing to do anything to please my new best friend. And my anorexia was proud of me.

The arguments about food were the first times that Anorexia actually interacted with my family. (It was almost as if she was talking through me.) But they didn't know – and would never know – how brilliant she was. We were a perfect team.

The more I began to rebel, the easier it got to avoid mealtimes. I would go out for hours in the evenings, sneak into clubs with my friends and spend hours with different boys. Maybe I was still looking for self-worth. Or maybe I liked the sense of achievement. I just remember feeling so wanted when Anorexia came into my life, and it was the same when guys came on to me. On some level, I knew I was getting a reputation, but it didn't matter. I didn't care.

I knew my behaviour annoyed my parents, and that just made things easier for me. They just didn't know how to get through to me, so they left me alone and stopped trying to make me eat. There's a point when you just can't argue about the same things any more.

I wasn't afraid of getting told off. I was a long way past that.

One evening, when Kate had to come and pick me up, she found that I'd passed out in the street after going out drinking with a school friend.

My parents were furious. Of course they were. But it didn't bother me, so I did it more and more. I only really cared when my netball coach took me aside at the end of a game and told me that if I ever turned up for a game drunk or hungover, I would be off the team.

My other way of coping, apart from being out and about all the time, was to focus on others. For me, this meant rebelling even more and finding my self-worth with boys. I didn't feel worthy enough for anyone, so I became something that people would use. Whenever it got too much for me, I would just switch off or self-destruct so that they would leave. Over the next few years I became involved with one boy after another; ever since the sexual abuse my relationships had been strange. They'd been hard to understand and hard to appreciate. I self-destructed to protect myself, and chose boys that were all just as bad as each other. I stopped caring about me. I stopped thinking about my safety altogether. I would go out in the evenings and risk walking home alone in the middle of the night. I felt nothing at all, and I loved that.

If I ever felt weak, Anorexia gave me strength. I gave myself over to her, mind, body and soul. She was my most trusted friend; the only one who really mattered.

I didn't get hurt if boys messed me around anymore. I didn't cry when my parents argued. And if anyone else got too close to me, I would push them away. I was afraid that Anorexia would get jealous. She was in control now; she dictated my life. But I didn't mind that at all. We were inseparable friends and she knew best.

I still had a good, strong group of school friends around me who stuck by me through "thin and thinner"! Looking back, I know it can't have been easy for them. And I wonder how much they noticed. Did they ever realise something was wrong? Or was it a shock for them when I ended up in hospital?

Over that summer, I went out even more with my friends, so I was barely at home. I didn't eat, but I drank a lot. I was acting like a spoilt, rebellious child. I loved it when I got home to see that Mum had left the light on for me. But it was only later that I found out she'd lie awake for hours, waiting to go to sleep until she'd hear me come home. (More guilt!)

Sometimes I'd meet a guy in a club and go back to his place. We'd just lie there, kissing and talking, and then in the early hours of the morning, I'd head home, still drunk, across the Downs in the pitch-black. Maybe I actually wanted something to happen? Perhaps then I'd get some support. Or maybe I was just so detached from my emotions that I didn't care. Nothing seemed to scare me on those late walks home, and if I did ever feel uneasy, I would talk to my anorexia, and she would reassure me.

Wearing a mask was tiring, but I was good at hiding things. Really, I was a drunken, emotional mess, just pretending that everything was fine. Being silent seemed like the only option; it was certainly the easiest option. But in between the silences, I just wanted to rebel any way I could.

Mum had been funny about the idea of me having a big party for my sixteenth birthday. So, of course, I made sure I had one anyway! I got so drunk that I vomited everywhere, smacked my head on the outside step, and finally passed out on the sofa. What had I become? Was I trying to make myself feel something? Or was I just masking the pain because I couldn't channel it any other way? The morning after my birthday, I got up and went to Cheltenham for a singing competition. My head was pounding, but at least I was out of the house – and I didn't have to eat anything. Another little victory!

By this time, my mum had begun doing some outreach work in Bristol. They had a bus in the centre of town, providing hot drinks for homeless people on Friday and Saturday nights. One night I got drunk and turned up at the bus. It must have been so humiliating for her seeing me there, this loud, drunk, flirty, insecure girl – her daughter – who was wasting her life away. Waiting to die.

I was impervious to embarrassment now. My feelings were all locked up and inaccessible, except for one time when I got a reminder of what real emotion felt like.

I was halfway through getting dressed after getting back from a run when I got the phone call. It was my mum's number, but when I picked up, it wasn't Mum speaking. It was a man's voice. He spoke quickly and said he'd found Mum pulled over in her car. She had been sick and he'd called the paramedics.

Almost before he'd finished speaking, I was out of the house and on my way. I ran up Stoke Hill, across the Downs, and saw the car. Mum was bent over the steering wheel and Mollie was with her, tears streaming down her face, not knowing if Mummy was going to be alright.

I was terrified – such a razor-sharp sensation – but for Mollie's sake, I had to be strong. Dad came to pick up Mollie while I went with Mum in the back of the ambulance. I knew she'd been having problems with her heart, but I had been shut off from the fear, until now. Now, I was completely out of my comfort zone. I wasn't thinking about my anorexia; I was just giving into my feelings.

Was Mum going to die? I wanted to apologise for another argument we'd had about food the night before, but she was completely zoned out. When Dad joined us at the hospital, I knew I had to be strong for him and the family.

When I knew that Mum was going to be okay, the emotions started to switch off again. And I felt a different kind of guilt take their place. I had pushed Anorexia to one side and I was already thinking about how I could make it up to her. But I had a way. All I had to do was promise Anorexia that I would be her best friend, forever.

So I started to work even harder. I pushed my body to even greater extremes.

A friend gave me the idea of making myself sick after meals. Brilliant!

It was like a whole new way of beating my family and friends. This was a way of avoiding conflict between my anorexia and those around me. I could please everyone and no one would really know what was going on. After a meal, I'd make my excuses and head straight up to the bathroom for a "shower" after dinner. I always used the power shower; it was loud enough to drown out the sounds of vomiting.

I'd turn on the shower and turn up the radio. Then I'd kneel over the toilet and make myself vomit. It was horrible and uncomfortable at first. And it hurt. But every time, it got a little bit easier. I found that downing water at the same time helped the food to come up more easily. And soon it was just a routine part of my day.

I was almost scientific about it; studying the food that came out, trying to make sure that I'd thrown it all up. If not, I'd make myself vomit some more until there was only water coming up; sometimes there'd be blood. And that was really frightening. But I knew I had to keep going with it.

My new routine still wasn't enough for me. For a minute or two, when I'd flushed it all away, I'd lose the disgust with myself for eating the calories, but I knew it was only a short-term gain.

I had to do more. Sitting cold and naked on the floor, I'd look down at myself with the same hatred and revulsion.

After an hour or so in the bathroom, I'd finally shower and wash the vomit out of my hair. Then I'd clean my teeth and crawl into bed. Empty, lost and drained of all energy, I hated having to make myself sick, but it seemed like the only way to please my family and my anorexia. But who did I want to please more? I didn't know any more. If I ever began to feel guilty about making myself sick, I would pull myself together and focus on the fact that it was probably my parents' fault anyway. It was simple: they made me eat, so they made me want to be sick. If they didn't interfere, it wouldn't have happened.

I was worried about the effect that being sick every day was having on my teeth. The acid erosion was taking its toll. I'd read about it all, of course. I knew everything there was to know about my "condition". And now I was starting to think that maybe they were right; maybe there really was something wrong with me.

But as soon as I began to doubt myself and what I was doing, my anorexia came back in full force, reassuring me I was doing the right thing. So, I just carried on. What other choice did I have? When no one else understood, she "got" me completely. So, I put my trust in her absolutely.

That summer, we headed off to the New Wine Trust summer camp with our church, as always. I loved the social side of it; my friend Charlotte and I would plan our outfits weeks in advance. Because it was a safe environment, Mum was relaxed, and let us roam around until all hours on the campsite. There were plenty of boys about, and I loved all the male attention, thrived off it almost. And if my friends didn't like it, what did it matter? I just boxed up the niggling sense that I'd let them down and got on with it.

The food had never really been a problem until that year. Mum was making a big issue out of it, and I was finding it harder to avoid mealtimes. One evening, I knew we were all going to have chips with Charlotte, but I figured out a solution. After eating,

I'd just have to "go and shower in preparation for the evening". Everyone would be happy and no one would suspect a thing.

As I threw up chips in the shower, I knew I'd managed to keep everyone happy. Well done, me! But something was wrong – the sick wouldn't flush down the plughole. The panic nearly overwhelmed me. How was I going to hide this?

There was no one waiting to use the other showers, so I threw my clothes over the top of the next shower cubicle and slid underneath the gap, leaving my shower locked. It was hard sliding under the door, with the cold, damp floor rubbing over my skin, but I didn't care. I felt no shame or guilt until I came out and saw Charlotte standing there. She wanted to know why the door was locked, but I didn't know what to say, so I made up some silly excuse. After what felt like ages, I managed to persuade her to leave the showers, and slightly disgruntled, she headed back with me to our tent. That was the closet I had ever got to being caught. And it terrified me.

There had been the usual flings that summer – classic Hope Virgo behaviour – but then I met Andy. And it felt different. We even decided to meet up after New Wine. He came to see me in Bristol, and I stayed with him in Milton Keynes. He was lovely, but definitely not allowed to meet Anorexia. I knew I had to be "normal" if I wanted to keep seeing him and I had to try to hide all my eating habits.

Maybe it was at that point that I thought that maybe there really was something wrong with me. It hadn't really occurred to me before, but I suddenly felt embarrassed, maybe even ashamed of making myself sick.

A couple of months after my seventeenth birthday, I ran my first half marathon. I completed the thirteen miles in under one hour and forty minutes. I hadn't eaten anything for four days! Now that's an accomplishment, isn't it? It felt so amazing. I was absolutely on top of the world, invincible. I bet no one else had run it that quickly, having had so little food.

I couldn't find Mum afterwards. Later she told me she'd been too scared to watch. She knew by then that my body was under too much pressure, and thought I might actually have collapsed and died on the way round. But her fear didn't really register with me. I just remember thinking how amazing it was that you could push your body so hard. I couldn't quite believe how much my body could take. That realisation was exhilarating. And it was terrifying.

CHAPTER 5

BEING WATCHED

Caroline Virgo, Hope's mum:
It was the school that first raised real concerns about the drop in Hope's weight, and it was a massive shock. Obviously, we'd noticed how slim Hope had been getting, but anorexia? That simply wasn't in our comprehension.

I took Hope to see her GP after the school intervened. At that time, the GP didn't seem to understand anorexia any better than I did. But thanks to pressure from the school, he gave us a referral letter for the Children and Adolescence Mental Health service (CAMHs).

While we were waiting for an appointment, Hope's weight suddenly plummeted. Three weeks after seeing the GP, we knew we needed an appointment urgently. I made calls, the school made calls, and, at last, we were given an immediate appointment.

Hope:
From the time I was referred to CAMHs, I knew I was being watched. Until then, I'd got away with it. Anorexia had helped me stay one step ahead of everyone else. But now, they were on to me and I knew I was going to have to up my game. I still didn't know why everyone was interfering. It was my life. Why couldn't they just leave me alone? Why didn't they accept the fact that

that voice in my head was the one thing that was making me so happy?

On my first trip to CAMHs, I had no idea what to expect. But I knew I had a one-hour session to suss everyone out, find out what the weigh-in plans were, and most of all, try to convince everyone that nothing was wrong.

I arrived with my mum and we sat in silence in the small, dingy waiting room. The kid sitting opposite me looked weird. I looked around some more. Everyone looked weird. I didn't belong here. There'd been a mistake. I was normal. Wasn't I?

I watched the people come and go, and passed the time making up little stories about them all. The boy opposite me, shaking in his seat, had definitely killed someone ... his dad first and then his younger brother. Maybe they were trying to blame his brain so he didn't have to go to juvenile prison. Sitting next to him, his mum looked scared. Maybe she thought she was going to be next on his kill list. Maybe she would be ... or maybe she was secretly pleased he had killed her husband.

Another teenage girl looked angrily around the room, cuts all over her arms. So she was self-harming, but why? Maybe she had been abused? I watched her and wondered what made her tick, why she hurt herself like that. And I wondered if she had a best friend in her mind who encouraged her to cut herself ...

'Jennifer Hope Virgo!' The call of my name cut through the silence in the room. Mum gave me a reassuring look and we were shown into a messy office, with thank you cards pinned to the walls. I was itching to get away. I had far too much to be getting on with.

The appointment was a bit of a blur – Mum talked a lot about our family and said that Dad wasn't engaged with our life. They wanted to know about my feet too; they were covered in cuts and blisters and my nails were black. I knew they were just a bit sore from all the running, but they seemed to think they should be healing faster.

And then I got weighed. I can't remember what weight I was, but I remember they weren't happy. They told me I had to put on a lot of weight, fast.

They went on and on about "next steps". But I remember telling them they were blowing it all out of proportion. So, I'd lost a lot of weight, but it definitely wasn't too much. How could it ever be too much?

I got a score of forty-four on the Eating Attitudes Test (EAT-26). I know from the anorexia forums that some girls were getting even higher scores than that, but the "experts" say that if you score over twenty, you need further evaluation. So, officially, I was a case for treatment.

After the appointment, we received a huge summary of everything that had been discussed. These were some of the highlights:

"We offered Hope an urgent appointment ... Hope is a seventeen-year-old girl who presented with at least a four- to five-month history of severe anorexia nervosa with a restricting pattern with marked self-induced vomiting as a weight loss strategy ... Hope had responded to our concerns about her damaged feet which are not healing by seeing a nurse today and the GP practice has agreed to run blood tests to ensure there are no physical complications ... We have discussed a general pattern of support and encouraged Hope to start taking small regular meals if necessary using high calories liquid preparations (I prescribed a small supply of Ensure Plus) ... Hope's bloods indicate that her K (Potassium) has been low (3.2) ... she has agreed with the cooperation of her GP surgery to have her K checked weekly ..."

At this point I wasn't actually sure there was anything the matter with me. I had this voice in my head that told me what to do, but so what? As long as I was happy and it was making me happy, surely that was all that was wanted. Why couldn't they leave me alone? And come on. Anorexia?! I was definitely not thin enough to be anorexic!

Dad didn't come to the first session, so the letters were changed to give his account of things. Mum and Dad blamed each other for so much. And it upset me that everyone was trying to blame someone else. I didn't think there was any point; my attitude was one of "these things happen". Perhaps that was just because I didn't want to give in to the emotion, or take on any responsibility.

I could see that Dad was hurting so much, could see the disappointment on his face. Maybe I really had failed everyone.

And then it began. The never-ending round of CAMHs visits, being weighed at every opportunity, the endless conversations and questionnaires. Hearing doctors telling me I was going to die.

I remember the awkwardness of family therapy, of Mum, Dad and the five of us sitting in a room with a family therapist, trying to achieve some reconciliation, or perhaps some answer that'd make everything alright. If it hadn't been so serious, it would have been comical.

Kate tried hard to say things, but mostly we ended up sitting in silence. I felt so bad for putting Mollie and Samuel through it all. Mollie was so young, and Samuel looked as if he had shut his emotions off completely. Mum and Dad spent those sessions bickering, trying to put fault on someone else.

Mum collected me for my CAMHs appointments every other Thursday at 2.15 pm. Registration after lunch finished at 2.05 pm, so when everyone else went off to their next lesson, I had ten vital minutes to water-load. I'd head straight to the locker room where I had stashed away four two-litre bottles of water. I would then spend the next ten minutes downing water. I would bloat and pile on pounds in water-weight, getting more and more dizzy as stars flashed before my eyes. But I knew it was worth it. I knew I had to trick them.

As the water-loading got harder, I'd stuff weights in my pockets so it would look like my weight was continuing to go up. It was all going brilliantly. Month by month, it looked like I was gaining weight. I would layer up with leggings, hoodies and trackies – so many pockets to hide so much in! It was all going wonderfully. With help from Anorexia, I was outsmarting them all. It meant that I could then sit in my therapy sessions saying, 'I'm fine! Life's fine. Everything's fine!' and no one had to know the truth. I had created this win-win situation for everyone involved.

But then, one afternoon Mum was early, and I didn't have time to water-load. In a mad panic, I left the weights in my locker at school. I was so afraid that they'd find out I'd been lying all this time. Would they be stricter now? I sat in the car next to Mum, sweating, anxiety spreading through my whole body.

I still had a chance. Maybe there'd be time when I got to the hospital. I could go to the bathroom and drink out of the tap. My mind was racing. We'd been doing so well, but now I had let Anorexia down. I had failed my best friend. Why had Mum been early? She was never early!

We arrived at the hospital, and after trying to drink water out of a tap and failing, I walked into the appointment and within seconds was weighed. It showed that I had dropped more than ten kilograms in just one week.

I made my feeble excuses. But I knew I had to try harder. The next week was a nightmare, and to top it off, I got told I was no longer allowed to drive. I lost all my independence, but instead of using this as a reason to get well, I used it as a reason to turn more and more people against me. With Mum watching my every move, I did whatever I could to sneak food into my pockets at mealtimes. The sloppy mess of whatever was on my plate would seep through my pockets and dribble across my skin, feeling cold and clammy.

I had to work harder than ever now. I got more tips from dieting sites and anorexia forums. The forums were great for sharing ideas and motivation. I'd been avoiding eating as much as possible, but now that they were on to me, I knew I couldn't get out of every single meal.

One evening I got back late and Dad told me I had to have a snack. I was furious. I argued with him, I shouted at him. But Dad wasn't budging. It was so unlike him. He was normally such a pushover; normally I could steamroller through any objections. So I angrily started stuffing myself with toast and then shouted, 'Is that enough?'

I looked straight into his eyes as I flung the rest of the bread across the floor. His eyes were filling with tears, but I didn't care. He had been mean. He had made me eat when I didn't want to. He didn't understand. I stared awkwardly at him and then went straight up to the bathroom, where I spent the next hour or so vomiting, downing water, vomiting, downing water, bringing up blood … Then the old, familiar cycle of feeling empty and alone took over. I crawled into bed, not knowing how I would have the energy to face another day.

As my parents got stricter with me, I had to make myself sick more often. I was so fed up; it was their fault my teeth were bad. When I went to the dentist, I felt so nervous in case my breath smelt or there were bits of vomit stuck in my teeth. Jackie, the dentist, started counting my teeth and doing her regular checks. Then she asked to do an x-ray. I was confused and Mum looked stressed. This wasn't normal procedure.

The x-rays showed the acidic erosion on my teeth. They were crumbling.

Jackie asked if I was drinking lots of fizzy drinks, but before I had time to answer Mum jumped in. 'She makes herself sick.' I was furious with her. I immediately denied it and got upset. I was so angry with Mum. She didn't get it at all. No one did.

Jackie immediately defused the situation and explained what dental work she'd need to carry out to help my teeth survive. I guess for once, Anorexia was wrong and Google was right. My body *was* falling apart.

I climbed into the back of the car, feeling sad, alone and furious. I stared out of the window, shutting off from the rest of the world, and I talked to Anorexia. I was comforted by her closeness to me. She reassured me it would be okay. She told me she would teach me new ways of not eating. I knew she would.

I trusted her. She wasn't going to reject me or suddenly leave me. She was with me for life.

Mum tried to talk to me as I got out the car, but I wanted nothing to do with her. I headed upstairs to change before going out for a run.

I had met a wonderful boy over the summer called Andy. He was few years older than me and shortly after we got together, he went to university. I quickly slipped back into the same spiral of self-destructive behaviour. After a few weeks I went to see him in Loughborough. I had already started CAMHs and was being watched like a hawk at home, so I couldn't wait to get away from my family. But when I got off the bus, he looked at me like he didn't even know me. I barely ate any more and was just about too tired to care. I felt nothing. We still managed to have a nice weekend together, but we didn't talk about food. I guess he couldn't face the reality that the girl he was sort of dating was slowly withering away before his eyes. And however much he cared about me, I didn't care about anything apart from pleasing Anorexia.

Looking back, I often wonder what he saw or what he thought when he looked at me. Could he ever have understood what was going through my mind? We would lie in his bed, talking about his day and what he'd done, but my mind was so unfocused, it would just wander back to exercise and calories. With me around, Andy didn't exactly have the best freshers' week experience, but I was selfish back then. I didn't even care if his worry for me was eating him up from the inside.

The girl he had fallen for over the summer had gone. Instead he was left with an empty, emotionless shell.

Would he still feel the guilt of breaking up with someone who was dead inside?

CHAPTER 6

SPIRALLING OUT OF CONTROL

Caroline Virgo, Hope's mum:

Hope's issues with food had originally been thrust into the limelight in such a dramatic way nine months previously. It had all happened after Hope decided she wanted to be confirmed at our church. She invited her boyfriend at the time, a friend of her elder sister's, Yusef. It was agreed that he would have Hope's room and she would sleep in the spare room. But she had left her diary under the pillow ...

Yusef read her diary. He told Kate, who then told me. We talked to Hope and she assured us that we could remedy it. It took me nine months to realise that we couldn't.

Those nine months were hard work. I had to try to prepare food she would eat, but I also had to maintain some sort of normality in a very busy household. I'd set up a charity around that time, which suddenly became very busy too. It was getting harder and harder to juggle all my responsibilities.

Hope's behaviour around food became more disordered. She began to cook sweet, fatty food for her brothers, and every time she made a terrible mess. On the worst occasion, I came home to find the kitchen completely trashed. There was food debris everywhere and an overturned plant pot. Sitting in the middle of the congealing food mess was the new puppy that Hope had let into the kitchen.

I tried my best to protect my other children from what was happening. I was ignorant of the concept of an eating disorder. It just seemed like a phase Hope was going through – something that would sort itself out in time. Little did I know that Hope would get so unwell and come so close to dying.

Hope:

I was tired. I no longer had the energy to stand in a locker room, downing water. I had failed at water-loading before my last trip to the hospital (the second time I had done this in my whole five months at CAMHS) and I'd lost the will to do it again.

On my next trip to the hospital, my weight hadn't budged at all. I was given protein shakes which were full of fat and calories, and told I had to drink three a day! I looked at the dietary information: 330 calories in one tiny carton! As soon as we got out of the pharmacy, Mum got me to drink one. I didn't know what to do or say. The thought of drinking it didn't just make me feel sick, it made me feel disloyal to Anorexia.

But I didn't have a choice. I think part of me was scared that the doctors had been right – that my heart could stop at any moment.

That evening, after I'd managed to force down two of the drinks, Anorexia shouted at me. She told me I had to pull myself together or I would fail at this as well. She was right. No one knew what I was trying to do, and everyone was just trying to make me fat, just because they didn't have the same willpower or determination to diet. They were jealous.

I kept all the cartons in my cupboard. I took them out and tried to work out if there was any way to get the content out without having to drink it! Ideas swam through my head …

Come on Hope! You're clever, you're resourceful, you need to work this out!

After about thirty minutes, I had it! I thought that if I could unseal the foil bit where the straw went in, I might just be able to switch the contents for water, and then glue the lid back on!

The first carton was quite hard to do, and I had to be really quiet so no one would hear my trips to and from the bathroom. But after the first few I got into a routine: unseal it, pour the liquid into a spare bottle, empty it, re-fill with water, then re-seal.

I stayed up for hours to do every single carton. I was literally a genius. The next day I sat with the deputy head teacher, happily drinking water out of my carton. I had succeeded in tricking her and everyone around me. I felt so smug and no one ever knew why. What a win! But in reality, Anorexia – my best friend – had turned into a manipulative bitch. She was slowly destroying me and ruining everything around me. But I couldn't see it. If I ate, I felt horrible. If I didn't eat, I felt great! So why would I choose to keep eating?

The lies and deceit carried on. I lost more weight but made excuse after excuse. I told everyone at CAMHs I was fine. But whenever I said that, my doctor would look at me and say, 'Do you mean fine? Or "fine" as in fucked up, insecure, neurotic and emotional?' I would always laugh awkwardly, not entirely sure how to respond.

Of course, he was right. I was anything but fine. But it didn't feel like my problem. They were making me believe there was something dramatically wrong with me, when really, I just wanted to lose a little bit of weight.

As I ate less, I lost the energy to fight my anorexia. At times I wanted to fight, but I just couldn't do it. I was lost, trapped in this vicious cycle. It seemed like Anorexia was my best friend, but was she? Did she even really care? There were evenings when I would absolutely hate that voice in my hate. I just wanted it to stop telling me what to do.

I would battle with myself at every mealtime. Was it better for me not to eat and feel bad, or eat and feel worse? At mealtimes, I would watch my family watching me as I pushed the food around my plate, accidentally dropping bits on the floor and filling my pockets with it. But it was getting harder. Everyone was watching and waiting for my weight to go up. Instead, it continued to slip down, and it was getting harder and harder to hide it.

Mum would get phone calls if I ever went to the gym, which made working out even harder. I was cross with everyone around me – cross at them for interfering, cross that people I didn't really know were helping my parents instead of helping me. I wanted everyone to leave me alone. Most evenings I would gobble down some vegetables and refuse to eat anything else. Then I'd down litres of water, run upstairs to my bedroom, pull out a bin bag and make myself sick. I couldn't escape the stench of vomit. It crept out of my room and followed me everywhere.

One evening I vomited so much I was sick all over the carpet. I turned off the lights, pretended to be asleep, and spent hours trying to clean it. Then I switched on YouTube and ran on the spot for hours, trying to distract myself from the pain by watching endless, unfunny videos, while Anorexia shouted at me. Nothing I did was good enough for her any more. As the sweat dripped down me, she told me I was failing and that she was very unhappy with me.

In the early hours of the morning, smelling of sweat and vomit, I crawled into bed and cried myself to sleep. I knew that in just two hours' time, I would wake up again and face the day, knowing that everything would be just the same. I didn't know how long I could keep going. I just wanted to die. My life was spiralling out of control. I hated Anorexia more than anything in the world but felt unable to do anything about it. Every night I would lie in bed telling myself that tomorrow I would just start eating again, that somehow everything would be okay. But the next morning I would get up, look in the mirror, weigh myself and be back on it with the Anorexia, telling myself that I would just do one more day.

The week before I went into hospital, Mum called in a frantic state. The results of my ECG were back, and showed that my heart was in a critical condition. They wanted me to go straight home, pack a bag and head to the hospital for a check-up. When I walked through the front door I didn't know if my mum was angry, sad or what. I wasn't even sure if I really believed her. They had told me this for months now that my body would eventually shut down, but the shock tactics never worked for me. Maybe this was just another one of these plans to make me eat.

I didn't know if I was angry or relieved that someone else was going to take over my fight. And I didn't know how it made me feel about my anorexia. Had she betrayed me, or had I let her down?

That night Mum served up tuna and a jacket potato with salad, and I stared at it as it stared back at me. 'Don't even think about eating that,' Anorexia whispered into my ear. 'It won't make you feel better.' I began to work it out – in total, this meal would be about 400 calories. But I reckoned if I moved quickly, I could sneak half the tuna into my pocket …

Success! 'Right, now, let's just eat half of what's left, and call it a day,' Anorexia said.

Everyone was tense, so Kate suggested going to the cinema to see *Ratatouille*. It seemed like a good distraction. We headed for the cinema, the tuna still in my pocket. How was I going to get rid of it? I wasn't even allowed to be on my own for a minute any more. There was no way for me to dispose of it, so I just had to sit through the film with my pocket smelling of tuna.

It was all worth it in the end. After the cinema, we drove home and I actually felt happy. I looked at Kate sitting in the car next to me. She was fantastic. I loved her so much. I'd really enjoyed our evening. We listened to silly pop music and reminisced about the old days. It felt … normal. Right up until we got home, anyway. I said goodnight to my parents and then went straight back into the nightly ritual of working out secretly in my room.

The next day, I went for my preliminary assessment at Riverside Hospital with Mum and Dad. I was seen by a nurse, a doctor and a psychologist. They weighed me, told me I was in a critical state and then showed me to a bedroom. After what felt like a lifetime, they came to a decision.

I was told I had to come back in the morning at 10.30 am. To stay.

I felt a bit lost. I was confused. I still didn't really believe anything was wrong. They were telling me I could die in the next two weeks. But I couldn't take it in. It made no sense. They didn't know me. They didn't know how strong I was.

I got home from the appointment and Mum didn't even see the point of trying to make me eat lunch. Maybe they'd officially given up on me. About bloody time!

I sat down at my desk and looked blankly at my homework. It barely registered. I looked around at the stains on the floor from where I had made myself sick, and I tried to think of a time when I had felt happy in this room.

Quite calmly, I got a bin bag and emptied drawers full of sick bags and half-empty food packets into it. I felt alone, isolated. I knew I had disappointed everyone, but I still didn't want to fight this. I couldn't – *wouldn't* – believe anything was really wrong. But one realisation hit me hard. I knew that it would be so much easier if I was dead – and it would be better to be dead than fat.

CHAPTER 7

HOPE VIRGO VERSUS THE WORLD!

Caroline Virgo, Hope's mum:
Anorexia is very destructive. The period before Hope went into hospital, I watched her completely losing control. And there was nothing I could do about it.

It was heartbreaking watching one of my children – who I loved and cared about so much – dying in front of my own eyes. And it was such a terrible feeling knowing that there was nothing I could do to help.

During that autumn, there were a few good days, memories to cherish. The days were crisp and golden and we walked together a lot. There were even some moments when she seemed so much more in control. She could still be reasonably objective about what was happening to her and how she was feeling. But I could feel the illness taking a tighter grip on her.

I wanted to watch her at mealtimes and afterwards, but I just couldn't. I had two younger children at home, and they needed my time and attention too. But I couldn't shake the horrible feeling of having to cope with the situation on my own. The hopelessness of it came to me full force one evening when I had been up to school to collect my son, and arrived home to discover that Hope was very audibly making herself sick. I think that was the watershed moment when I realised I couldn't keep Hope at home any longer.

I gave Hope an orchid when she went into hospital. I needed us both to feel like we had hope. So I chose a flower I thought would live for two to three months. I thought she'd be home before the flower perished.

But things didn't turn out like that at all ...

Hope:

It was 29th November 2007. I was seventeen years old.

I stood in the doorway of the hospital, my hair thinning, my skin yellow. I had no idea about the fight that I was about to embark on. It wasn't just a fight to get well; it was a fight to turn my life around, and save my life.

My care plan read:

Hope is a seventeen-year-old girl who presents with anorexia nervosa. She has been suffering weight loss for some time. She has also been attempting to control her weight with self-induced vomiting. Hope will be attending the unit as an in-patient ... At the time of her admission her BMI is below 15 ...

The care plan showed my short-term weight gain targets, an endless schedule of supervision after meals, and extended bed rests. Exercise was not allowed.

I read it over and over again. I didn't know what was wrong with having anorexia. And I certainly didn't understand how they expected me to eat and not want to run. Worse, I started to think about how I was going to hide food with so many nurses around.

I was told that this was stage one of the three-stage eating disorder programme. Stage one was for anyone with a BMI of 16 or under. Stage two, a BMI of 16–18.5, and stage three 18.5+. They told me the objective was for me to get to a healthy weight in the short term, and then in the long term, learn how to manage my weight day-by-day. They wanted me to get to a BMI of between 19 and 22. But I knew there and then that I would definitely not budge above 19. And I'd already begun thinking about how I would justify it when I got to that point. Luckily, I found out that they regarded 18.5 as a healthy weight at the adult unit down the road. So that made my decision for me: 18.5 would be my cut-off point.

My eyes scanned further down the page and fixed on directives like "No diet drinks", "No low-fat foods", "No chewing gum", "three meals and three supplements a day", "bed rest after each meal", "forty-minute limit for mealtimes" and "no calorie-burning posturing". Bloody hell! Could the rules be any stricter? I knew it was going to be tough to sneak food off my plate and sneak exercise into my schedule. But they hadn't reckoned with my resourcefulness. I was a pro! Anorexia and I would show them who was best.

That first day in the hospital wasn't how I had imagined it. In my mind, it had been a lot more like the movies: people shuffling around with white coats on and screaming weirdos being pinned down to tables. It wasn't like that at all. But even as I stood in the doorway on that first day, begging Mum to take me home, I was terrified of what was to come.

I was supposed to be at school studying for my A Levels, not stuck in a hospital. I wondered what people at school would think. What would they say about me?

The night before I had gone out to Pizza Express with my core group of friends. At the last minute they had all dropped their plans to come out for dinner, even though they knew full well I wouldn't eat anything. I had ordered a tuna salad with no dressing and I picked at it while making conversation. At that point none of what was about to happen felt like reality.

This was all so ridiculous and I still couldn't quite believe it. I was scared and worried about how much of life I was going to miss out on. Sixth form had been fun; I used to enjoy sitting around in the common room, watching endless episodes of *Friends* on television. And I knew that this school year, we were going to enjoy even more freedom. Or rather, *they* were. My friends were turning eighteen, going out more, meeting boys, drinking legally and enjoying their lives.

But me? I was stuck between four walls, restricted to life in hospital. I felt trapped and alone. I was scared none of the other girls would like me, and that I wouldn't fit in. I was scared that all my friends from school would lose contact with me and I would be forgotten. As I stood on the threshold of my new life, I was hit by a rush of emotions. I felt like I had no one to turn to now.

How had life come to this? How could my mum do this to me? Why was she giving up on me?

It was shocking how quickly my rigorously structured new hospital routine, became the norm. There was a crushing inevitability about it all ...

7.15 am: Get up and get weighed

We all had to queue up outside the medical room to be weighed. It was the most stressful way to start the morning.

Do you weigh more or less if you shower first?

Suppose the other girls overheard your weight?

What if it's gone up?

What if it's gone down?

All these questions and loads more ran through my mind every morning as I stood there, shivering in my underwear.

8.00: Breakfast

Breakfast consisted of 600 calories. Who starts the day with that much food?!

Breakfast was always tense as they pulled out the hospital bowls and everyone would pour milk and cereal, trying to get away with having as little as possible. (But if you didn't eat breakfast to their satisfaction, it just meant that staff would pour the cereal and milk for you, and spread thick butter and jam on toast.)

To help us gain weight more quickly, we had to start with full-fat milk. Yuck! We had to measure the milk up to the 200 ml line on a little plastic cup and drink it, before putting even more milk on our cereal. But if you were sneaky you could pour the drinking milk on your cereal instead. Weetabix was the best option. The milk soaked into the cereal, so the nurses couldn't dispute how much you'd had. It didn't matter whether or not I liked milk soaking into my cereal and making it soggy; I had no choice.

8.30: Eating Disorder Group

We had ED Group after every meal. We'd shuffle into the therapy room, pull up a cushion and sit awkwardly, looking down at the floor, waiting for someone to start with the age-old question, 'How did you find that meal?' Some days, if we were all fed up, we would sit for what felt like an age with no one saying anything.

9.00 – 11.00: Therapy, lessons or bed rest

Bed rest was prescribed if you were too unwell to do anything, or if you hadn't completed a meal. I spent my first month forced to have bed rest under supervision. I was watched constantly, so there was no chance of me exercising or trying to make myself sick.

But of course, I had my ways. When they were content that I was resting peacefully they'd leave me alone, and as soon as they were out of the door, I'd jump up and work out. It used to make me so proud when I beat the system like that!

11.00 – 11.20: Snack time

We all sat in the front room with different snacks. On my first morning I was given a high-protein, high-fat and extremely calorific drink. A nurse sat next to me, prompting me to drink it at regular intervals. And after a long twenty minutes, I managed one sip.

11.20 – 12.30: More therapy, lessons, bed rest or supervision

After snack time, I was taken up to my bedroom and a nurse sat outside my room while I was instructed to stay in bed until lunchtime. I lay there, trying to think about ways I could exercise. I was mentally exhausted and felt so lonely. I already hated being there. I was isolated, cut off from the world. My phone had been confiscated and there was no Wi-Fi, so I couldn't even use my laptop. My world had shrunk from school, friends, gossip and sports to almost nothing.

12.30 – 1.10: Lunch

13.10 – 13.15: ED Group

13.15 – 4.00: More therapy, lessons or bed rest

4.00 – 4.20: Snack time

Another 300 calories

4.20 – 4.30: End of the day

4.30 – 6.00: Visiting time/free time

At the end of my first day, the girls sat around my bed and we talked for ages before dinner. Anyone new coming in generated a mix of panic and interest. Would they be really skinny? Would they be nice? Would they co-operate with the system?

6.00 – 7.00: Dinner and ED Group

7.00 – 8.00: Visiting time/free time

8.00: Snack time
Another 300 calories

9.00: Lights out
There were four beds in my room. I shared with Sarah (anorexic) and Katy (anorexic), and Susan (OCD) was in a room on her own. It was quiet at that time of year, but it filled up quickly over the next few months.

Susan had been there the longest. She'd come in with a diagnosis of anorexia, but had since developed Control-OCD. Katy was on her second admission. It was handy having such pros around me; they knew how things worked, and were happy to answer all my questions about food. They told me I looked awful, which made me happy! The first few days were a blur of food, bed rest, tears and the occasional giggle with the girls in the evening.

Mealtimes were funny – I sat on my own and went through the same routine day after day – the food was served and I was prompted to eat, again and again by a long-suffering nurse. I could feel all the girls staring at me while I battled through it. We used to judge each other constantly, seeing who was eating what and who was managing to sneak any food away. It was draining. You had to have eyes in the back of your head, but I was learning. We were learning.

After three days, I was bored, tired and fed up. It was Friday night. Why was I stuck in hospital? At weekends, some of the other in-patients got to go home, leaving just two of us on the ward. My primary nurse was on the late shift, so she came up to see me before dinner. I was bored of being on my own in bed and I was glad to see her. She brought some huge pieces of poster paper with her and we stuck them together. First, she got me to draw myself as I imagined I looked. Then she drew around me – inside the outline I had drawn. It was only then that I realised that maybe, just maybe, I was seeing myself wrong.

I stared at the paper, lost for words. Why couldn't I see myself as being that small? Why did I feel so huge? After that she got me to stand in front of the mirror and look at myself. She put my hand on my bony shoulders and tried to make me think logically. It wasn't easy being so objective. But it was the first time that I'd been able to look at myself and see what others saw – if only for a moment.

CHAPTER 8

LEARNING TO LET GO

by Caroline Virgo (Hope's mum)

I vividly remember leaving Hope at the hospital. It felt like an acknowledgement that there was nothing more I could do to help her, and I was terrified. They were telling me my daughter might die. And they said that the survival rates for anorexia were lower than cancer.

We were all suffering. If your child is physically ill, you have a function as a parent, and you can still be a good one. Siblings can still be good siblings. But if your child has a mental illness, there is the double stigma of thinking that it's your own fault, as well as thinking that everyone else is blaming you. It is a very lonely place to be.

I knew it was hard on her brothers and sisters. Suddenly, however hard you try, the focus shifts to one child. I did what I could to contain the inevitable emotion that surrounded her admission, in order to protect the other children. Kate was away at university and James was in Australia, but Samuel and Mollie were still at home and it wasn't easy for them. Predictably, I tried to organise the household routine so that there was minimal disruption to the youngest two. I can't remember visiting times very clearly but I used to take things for Hope to do during visiting time, like cushions to sew. But most of all, I just remember how difficult it all was.

Even getting to the hospital was difficult. Because of the traffic, it could take an hour to get there, even though the unit was only a few miles away. Visiting time was strictly limited to an hour, so it all felt quite stressful.

Then there was the family therapy. I had to go with Hope's dad, and it was horrible. It seemed to me that Hope and her father were scapegoating me. The narrative seemed to be "You are the mother. You looked after her and she is ill, so it must be your fault". So many sessions ended with Hope telling me not to visit her again. She said she just didn't care. I was at a complete loss. I didn't know what I could do or say to help make things better.

We have spoken about it since, and Hope has acknowledged how difficult it must have been for me – but I guess that she will never understand just how hard it is until she has her own children.

And so time went on, with me still trying to do my best for everyone and planning life around hospital visits. I felt like the hospital must have had some faith in me as they allowed one of Hope's fellow patients to come to our house and stay over for New Year's Eve.

As the year passed, I fought to help Hope achieve her dream of going to university. I talked to the school and arranged for the teachers to go to the hospital to teach her. Emotionally, I had to work hard to let her go, to start giving her the independence that she would need to thrive at university. I knew I had to hold back and stop fussing over her. I only hoped that Hope didn't interpret this as indifference.

I had to learn how to cook the sort of meals "prescribed" by the hospital – and serve them, despite her protests. I also had to make decisions as to when it would be okay to let her go off and be a "normal" teenager, and when to make a judgement that it wasn't safe or appropriate. I even had to renegotiate relationships with friends' parents to make sure she had the support she needed when she was at their houses.

Our local vicar provided invaluable support and kindness too; he rang me on a regular basis and always had time to talk. He was an absolute star, and the one person with whom I felt I could say exactly what I wanted to.

I would also like to acknowledge the enormous kindness of her employers. Hope had had a Saturday job at White Stuff for at least a year when she went into hospital. To my absolute amazement, they continued to pay her sick pay (while she was in hospital) and held her job open for her (she did, in fact, return to work for them). This was an amazing act of kindness, and no doubt contributed to her recovery.

The taxi backwards and forward to the hospital, provided by the hospital, was also a massive help. Putting her in it in the morning allowed me some space from the rigid meal-focused regime and the continual stress of trying to do the right thing.

I will be forever grateful to the hospital. While it was a challenging year, and the therapy sessions were tough, I don't think that Hope could have survived without their support.

CHAPTER 9

PASTA AND CREAM CHEESE!

I counted myself lucky to be in a room with other girls. After lights out, we could sit up and chat for ages. We quickly learnt which nurses were strict and which ones didn't really seem bothered about late nights.

I knew that this would be my life for God knows how long, and I was afraid. I didn't think I'd have the energy to fight the system and go on facing this routine, day after day after day.

But I settled in pretty quickly in my first week. I liked most of the other young people in the hospital and I quickly learnt which staff to sit with at meals, and who I should avoid (mainly those who would give you more food, or who would push you to try and eat quicker).

Weekends in hospital were strange. And I was bored. My family came to see me and we sat awkwardly in the visiting room. The rest of the weekend was spent with the other in-patients watching television, playing pool, and sitting in the hospital corridors, making up stories. We weren't really allowed out in the grounds though, particularly if we weren't a specific BMI, so I felt quite trapped at times. It sucked hearing about all my friends from school going out and getting on with their lives. They were gradually turning eighteen, applying for universities, and I was missing out on everything.

Before the first week was over, I was told I had to start having full portions at mealtimes. I was furious. I hated the nurse who decided this, and I hated how quickly I was putting on weight. It was shooting up faster and faster and I couldn't control it. Each morning I would panic, unsure what to do. I felt horrific and I didn't understand why I had to keep eating.

A few weeks after I was admitted to the hospital, I began my sessions with Caroline. They were hard work but helpful, and they gave me the chance to talk about how I felt. They literally tried everything in there to try to keep us motivated. Most of us had cards with our key motivations on them. There were about ten on mine, which I carried around in my pocket – little inspirations like "I want to have children", "I want to travel", and "I want my life back".

I was beginning to learn that Anorexia hadn't really been my friend. She was a manipulative, selfish bitch, and she had destroyed me. She had made me think she was helping me, but she wasn't.

I had lost everything. I wasn't even able to enjoy my last year at school. I was stuck in a shitty hospital, being made to eat disgusting hospital food, and working through a rigid timetable, with my food being served up as if I was four years old. I shouldn't have been in hospital. I should have been out there living my life, drinking, clubbing, kissing boys ...

How had Anorexia convinced me to be her friend? It was her fault I was in this place. I hated her so much. And yet – as the days closed in, I climbed into bed and the chatter between my friends died down, I longed for her to hold me and tell me it would all be okay. Every night I promised her I would get out as soon as I could and lose all the weight again. I would be the girl she wanted me to be. The girl that she had become friends with. And we would go back to winning at life together.

Mealtimes with other anorexics can be a little bit of a minefield. Your eyes dart round everywhere, looking at what everyone else is having. You try so hard to focus on your plate, but can't help but feel distracted by what is going on. You compare every potato on your plate to see whether someone else's is bigger or smaller, watching what people are doing to not eat everything. It meant that arriving in a hospital and being lumped in with anorexic girls made the whole thing a bit more challenging.

About a month after I started, I began to talk more. By now, I was only being weighed every other day, which was so much better. One evening me, Katy and Susan were lying in our bedroom talking, when a nurse came round.

'You'll have to stay in your rooms for the rest of the evening. There's a new admission to the hospital tonight,' she explained.

None of us really knew what to expect, but after having our snack in our room, we put our pyjamas on and listened out. The sound of ambulance sirens got closer and closer, then the front door to the hospital opened and we heard the shouting. There was lots of banging and doors slamming, and then the hospital siren went off. Staff were running down the corridor. Dave (one of the nurses) came in after about an hour and a half to check on us. He explained that a very sick girl had arrived. The night continued like this: more shouting, hospital bells, staff running about until the early hours of the morning. At about 2 am Katy came and climbed into bed with me, and we huddled up close, reassuring each other that it would all be okay. We drifted off like that, and the next thing I remember, my alarm was going off again. It was 7.15 am and the daily slog of hospital began again.

When I went to the bathroom to have a shower, I saw that the sink had been half pulled off the wall overnight – I guess that explained the banging. After breakfast, we got our first glimpse of the new girl. She looked so spaced out. We were told we weren't allowed into her room until the staff let us. She was stuck in there and was only allowed out when no one else was around.

We only met her much later. We were watching television one evening when she came in. But she was still completely spaced out. I couldn't help but stare at her wrists, which were covered in cuts and scars. Later, she told us that she had been sectioned after she had tried to kill herself numerous times, and she had become quite violent. I really felt for her. I had only self-harmed a few times before and even then I hadn't been very good at it. I had cut my wrists with a razor. I'd just wanted to hurt myself, to make myself feel something. But it hadn't worked.

I had now been in the hospital for a few months and they wanted to restore some normality to my life by letting me go home for some meals at the weekend. Normality?! How was any of what I was going through normal? Nevertheless, one evening both my parents came in together for visiting time. They had specifically been asked to attend together to talk about the chance of me being allowed home for a few hours at weekends.

Chrissie, my primary nurse, talked us through it; I had to have my 300-calorie snack at home, and if I refused, my parents were to prompt me. *Good luck with that*, I thought. For some reason, I found it hard shouting at the hospital staff, but I knew that when I got home, it would be a whole lot easier to shout at my parents.

I was promised that if I ate my snack with my parents, I would be allowed home for three hours every weekend. So yes, I did it. Of course I did. I pretended it felt fine, even pretended that I loved every moment. I showed my parents that I was normal, but in reality, I was empty inside. I was aching.

I couldn't remember the last time my parents had seen me eat something without shouting or making a dash for the bathroom afterwards. They looked on, congratulating me as if I had just won a prize. I guess that, for them, it was a small accomplishment. They thought it was working, that I was "cured" and was starting to enjoy eating again. But I wasn't. I still loathed the thought of anything passing through my mouth, and my feelings of disgust after eating were just as real as ever.

I knew I wanted to go home, mainly to see Mollie (and to sneak some exercise in) so I ate it all up. On went my mask. It was "fine". A week later I went home for a trial meal. This was the next step to "normality" – why did they keep using that stupid word? They kept saying, 'Evidence shows that, if we do it like this, one day you will feel better.' What a joke!

I had no idea what to expect. We never ate meals as a family on a Saturday. I walked into the kitchen on that first Saturday back. Everyone was just standing around awkwardly. It was horrific; I felt like I was on show. And what did my bloody family make for me? Cream cheese and pasta!

I was livid. I couldn't believe I had to sit and eat it. I acted like a bratty child, picking my way through it while my nurse did her best to reassure me. What bollocks!

Going back home and seeing my bedroom with the stains still on the floor brought it all back to me – all the memories and all the pain. I just wanted to get out. I felt like I was back in a place where no one really understood me. I was trying, I really was ... but I knew I needed someone with me at all times now, someone who could appreciate what I was going through. Someone who would tell me to eat and help me reduce the guilt.

At the time, I was so cross with my mum for picking such a hard meal. (Now I'm glad to say we can look back and laugh about the crème fraiche incident!)

After that I was allowed to go back for occasional day trips, but they always felt so strained. No one really knew how to act around me. Everyone was on edge, and as soon as I went to the bathroom, I'd hear someone pacing outside. Was this really what my world and my life had become?

Alice joined the centre in December – another anorexic to add to the list. (Or, if Anorexia was feeling active, another competitor.) She was so sweet and so young when she arrived. I liked her away from the dining room, but loathed her when we ate. She would cut her food up really small, mash it around her plate, and hide bits in her yoghurt pot. Why did I hate her for that? Perhaps because she was doing a better job at beating the system than I was.

We all had our silly little tricks, but did they really make any difference to our weight? It still felt amazing to miss the odd calorie here and there. And every time I got away with it, I felt incredibly proud.

As December progressed, my weight continued to go up. I had done more therapy, but I still wasn't allowed to do any exercise. I had a heart-to-heart with Susan who told me I had to keep going. She said there was no point messing about and not eating, and there was no point in giving up, or they wouldn't ever let me out.

Just before the new year, Laura joined the centre. She was another anorexic; a nice, quiet girl. And she was super skinny. She mostly kept to herself, but she was good to be around. I only saw her get angry once, and that was with her nurse, John. I hated him as well; he was so gross and annoying. And he definitely didn't understand what we were all going through. Laura didn't really do things properly though – she pretended she was fine a lot of the time, but still cheated the system and always managed to get the smallest portions. But at other times she really came through. One evening Susan went to get a glass of water from the kitchen and discovered they'd changed the bread to a more calorific alternative. And it was thick sliced! We teamed up with Anorexia to get rid of it. We decided that Laura and Katy would distract the night staff, while Susan and I would get the bread.

It was scary creeping down to the kitchen, knowing that someone might find us. We waited for the signal, and then ran! We grabbed the bread but didn't know what to do with it, so we just threw it in the bin. What else could we do? We definitely didn't want it for breakfast.

Of course, all the staff knew, and it was recorded in the handover notes. But we didn't care. It was so worth it. Team Anorexic pulls together!

That evening, to celebrate, we had a proper girls' evening. We painted our nails, did our hair and make-up, and took photos of each other doing silly poses. It was one of my best nights in hospital – I actually felt like we were all really getting along. We laughed so much, told funny stories, and made a long list of the funniest things we'd heard in hospital, like the day we played Articulate and I described the word on the card saying: 'what we all have' and instead of saying anorexia Susan shouted out 'obesity!'

Looking back, that evening still makes me smile. But then, the next morning, the daily ritual of the weigh-ins and breakfast began again. Reality really sank in at breakfast when Laura "accidentally" sneaked some of her milk away by "spilling" it. It felt like the competition between us would never end.

What you have to understand is that a huge part of my illness was wrapped up in exercise. I exercised in dangerous ways to punish myself. When I was in hospital, I wasn't allowed to exercise at all. It was so hard. I felt trapped a lot of the time and completely unsure of what to do.

As I had done a lot of long-distance running before I got unwell, the hospital agreed for me to do this again, as part of helping me achieve some normality. But while it's so easy for others to start running again, for me it was a real challenge. Mandy, my nurse, offered to take me running a few times a week and it felt absolutely amazing when she did. I won't ever forget that first run – the wind in my hair, the feeling of my feet pounding the floor. I loved that feeling. What was amazing about Mandy is she taught me about the power of exercising in a positive way for our wellbeing. She listened to all my worries and questions. She helped me work out what I should be eating before and after a run. It was a complete game changer for me to be able to do this. It built up my confidence. It allowed me to really believe that I could do this, but it would take time.

CHAPTER 10

MY DIARY OF LIFE IN A
MENTAL HEALTH HOSPITAL

1st January 2008

Just saw Mum and I am so upset and angry at having to fight this so-called illness. My life is being ruined and it is so frustrating. I just want it all to go away, or to be left alone to do this my way. Being taken into hospital has ruined everything – my schooling, my relationships ... What if I am never actually well enough? What if everyone thinks I am okay and I am not? What if all this hard work crumbles and I am left fighting forever?

2nd January 2008

I have taken huge steps in weight gain and I'm doing well, but I feel so bloated and ugly. And there is still such a long way to go. Caroline still says I look dreadfully underweight (is that a good thing or a bad thing?). At least I'm getting better at talking about things. Someone new came into the unit today – her BMI is around 15. It's funny, when I was that thin, I never thought I looked that bad. But if she does, I must have done too.

I spent some time this evening looking at my motivating cards. I want to go to uni, to travel, to run again, so I have to get well. Right, tomorrow is a new day and I am going to start afresh.

3rd January 2008

I had a good chat with Hannah about my achievements so far

and yes, I know, I will eventually have to put on the weight. But that doesn't make it any easier. Why has this suddenly got so much harder? My BMI is still only 16.7 which, by definition, is underweight. Maybe I like being underweight?

I tried something new today and it felt good. I realised that if I am speedy in the bathroom, I can run up and down 50–100 times. If I do this whenever I go that will definitely help burn some calories and slow down the weight gain. I am desperate to see Mum even though we seem to fight quite a bit.

4th January 2008

Food was tough today – I feel so fat all the time. But I know that if I start letting Anorexia win again, the last few months will have been a complete waste of time. I hate that putting on a tiny bit of weight seems so terrifying. At least I'm fighting; Lizzie went back to stage one of the recovery plan today. She is so selfish! I hate people who don't try to fight this.

5th January 2008

Mum said I was looking good and not very underweight! What? I still have so much more weight to put on!

6th January 2008

Andy and I seemed to be back on track today. Our only hiccup was when we went to Sainsbury's to get some Frusli bars as snacks. They didn't have the ones I normally got so Andy suggested the other ones. But they had ten more calories in! We had a scene and he looked so upset with me. Anorexia never embarrasses me like that.

7th January 2008

Kate and June came in to see me today, and it felt a bit more normal. Although I wonder if this is ever going to be normal? They helped calm me down after the semi-skimmed milk ran out at breakfast and I had to have full-fat milk. Maybe distractions after meals are the way forward? I went back to my room after visiting hours and was still cross with Katy for finishing the semi-skimmed milk. Argh! I just feel so horrible. And it's weighing day tomorrow. I know I was happier when I was thinner, but I have to get well so I can get out of this never-ending nightmare.

8th January 2008

My weight went up today. But my motivation has deserted me. Susan and I managed to not put any milk in our cereal. Didn't even care how cross all the other girls were about it.

I HATE MY ANOREXIA SO MUCH! SHE IS A NASTY MANIPULATIVE BITCH WHO IS DETERMINED TO RUIN MY LIFE.

12th January 2008

I went home for the weekend – it was nice, but hard work. Someone had been in my room and taken all my calorie books. I didn't know where they'd gone, but was too scared to ask as I didn't want an argument with Mum.

13th January 2008

Back in hospital and I got in such a state over my evening snack. The tears welled up out of nowhere and I didn't know what to do. I hadn't felt anything for months, not even when I was really sick and struggling to deal with all the emotions.

I think the next plan is to sustain my BMI at 17 for a few weeks. I feel like the weight has gone on far too fast and my mind isn't keeping up or coping with it.

According to some of the nurses, most people with an eating disorder get into a rut at this point in their recovery. What a generalisation! And what do they really know? They haven't had anorexia; they can't understand it simply by studying it!

20th January 2008

I made myself sick tonight and sneaked half my dinner and snack away. And now I feel awful for doing it! Anorexia used to make me feel so good, but now she is being mean because I am putting on weight, and then when I listen to her, she doesn't even praise me any more. I just feel completely guilty.

23rd January 2008

I am so fed up of being in hospital and I am missing out on so much. Some of the girls from school came in tonight, which was fun, and YAY, they said I still looked super skinny! WOOOO!

25th January 2008

I got in trouble again today! First, they make me eat this disgusting food and then they stop me putting any salt on it – I only do it so I can't taste it. For God's sake, isn't it enough that I'm eating?! I am trying so hard, but my hair is still falling out, and I still have gross bits of hair on my body because I'm still underweight.

30th January 2008

The days are just merging into one long battle with my anorexia ... I'm trying to think about people in hospital that I find inspiring. The first one is definitely Susan. She managed to get over her anorexia (although now she's dealing with her OCD) but she seems to be doing so well. I'm fascinated that she can live her life and know just what to eat.

In my sessions, we've been talking about why I thought I had anorexia. My parents had always said it was down to the sexual abuse. I wasn't sure, but maybe it was linked; maybe I thought it made me less attractive. Anorexia felt like an achievement. I was so good at it! It even helped bring my family together. Now I don't know 100% if I want to get better ... is there any point?

31st January 2008

A new resolution – I am going to stop exercising. It's going to be tough, but I need to do something!

I cried when I had fruit and ice cream today, which seemed like such a setback. I still think about food 90% of the time. Maybe I am too hard on myself, but it isn't exactly easy battling my anorexia. Susan says I still look underweight.

Tomorrow they are bringing in new bowls – how am I going to know how much to put in? I want to have children so badly, and am constantly battling with myself on whether the exercise is worth it ... The death rate for anorexia is quite high and I know I don't want to die. Not yet! I need to get well – I want someone to love me, and someone to love. That could be another motivation to stay well.

1st February 2008

I was allowed out for a night – Mum and Dad trusted me to go to the Prom to watch Maeve's dad's band. It was so much fun, and although I didn't drink, I did feel normal for a change. I even met a boy! He was lovely and invited me out for lunch on the Monday, which is obviously pretty impossible as I will be back in hospital first thing tomorrow.

My weight is creeping up. I hope things get easier when I have put on all the weight I have to, and then I can just eat what other people eat ... or get out of here. And not eat.

Hit a bit of a brick wall this week and I covered all my food in salt to make myself suffer even more as I was eating it. It felt like I was letting Anorexia back in.

6th February 2008

The only positive about hitting a BMI of 17.5 is I can join the dance group this week. I thought about the future today. Am I ever going to be happy with my weight, or will I always think I'm fat? How do I know what to eat every day if I don't calorie count everything? I wish my mind would catch up with my physical changes. Lunch was okay, but really only because I had caused such a scene at breakfast and felt bad for the other girls. Susan keeps reminding me that however fat I feel now, it wasn't as if I felt any better when I came in.

10th February 2008

Dad says I still look very skinny and that the final bit of weight won't make any difference – here's hoping he's right. But I do still wonder, why me? Why did I get sick? Or is it just a weird phase? Will I ever feel better? Or is it genetic? Am I going to feel like this my entire life?

Do I like being anorexic? She is my best friend. She makes me numb to my feelings, but then she makes me feel rubbish, and technically, she is killing me ...

12th February 2008

Helen came in tonight. Was good to see her, although her first comment was, 'You look meaty!' Is that better or worse than people saying, 'You look well'? Hmm.

Charlotte got re-admitted today. She didn't do well enough, so she came back. What a shitty cycle to get in – maybe anorexia is a life sentence. Or maybe you can learn how to be underweight, hold it there, and somehow stay best friends with Anorexia and stay out of hospital.

In my therapy session, Caroline made me get angry with Steve for everything he had done. It was hard, but I lost control and then it all came out. I got in such a state, and I'm still not sure if it made me feel better or worse.

19th February 2008

I made myself sick after dinner tonight. I no longer get supervised after meals so I get a bit more freedom, but Emma heard and came and knocked on the door. I wouldn't let her in but she looked so disappointed in me when I came out. She really doesn't get it. She doesn't understand what it is like to have a best friend like Anorexia. You just don't know when she is going to creep up on you and urge you to exercise, make yourself sick, or avoid meals.

22nd February 2008

Period is back.

I feel awful.

Fat. Overweight. Whale-like.

I need to act fast so my weight drops!

7th May 2008

As my eighteenth birthday has crept up on me, I've been getting more and more scared. The unit has agreed to keep me on condition that I don't start losing weight. I guess that does help my motivation, but I know that if I lose it now, I'll be moved to an adult ward where they'll use the feeding tube and there'll be less support.

8th June 2008

James and Kate came back today. It is lovely seeing them both, but I feel like they're looking at me and thinking I am huge. Kate is so thin! It's horrible how fat I am. That's just something else she is better at than me. It is so unfair.

It's so hot, I have to wear summery clothes so I don't overheat, and that makes me feel even more grotesque next to her. I feel like everyone looks at me and thinks she's the thin one, the better anorexic, and I am just this fat person who is eating too much and shouldn't even be in an eating disorder ward.

There is always something telling me that if I lose weight, I'll be happier. Life will make more sense. Right now, the only thing stopping me is the fact I am getting weighed. I really don't feel like I am going to be able to cope next year on my own. I hate feeling all this emotion; it scares me. The only way I can stop from breaking down in front of everyone is by resorting to all the same behaviours – by disappearing upstairs or exercising. Although I am making up the calories, I still feel unable to go a day without running or going to the gym.

I keep trying to think about how sad I was when I was ill and how it ruined my life, but giving in to Anorexia still feels like the only way I have of feeling as if I'm worth something. If it feels so bad, why does it make me feel so good?

28th June 2008

My weight dropped today by 1.4 kg. I know it wasn't a lot, but it felt good and gave me a real feeling of comfort. But I know I have to keep going because if I slip now, then the last however-many months will have been wasted. And I don't want that. Something deep down inside me is helping me get through this.

30th June 2008

I went to see Grandma today. I hadn't really prepared myself for what awaited me: an emaciated woman I didn't even recognise. Her face was hollowed out. The warm smile was gone. If it hadn't been for the name above the bed, we wouldn't have known it was her. She knew she was going to die, but she didn't care. She had been consumed by the drive to lose weight. Was she winning by being thin?

Even at my lowest weight, I still feel obese. I can only presume it's the same for her, the idea that she would only be perfect when she was thin enough to die. It is so frustrating. Why has she done this to herself? How can she just let herself die? I am so angry with her for giving up.

Is that what people think about me? Do they feel that same frustration?

As I looked, I saw my future. But I don't want to be that person, lost and alone, wasting away in hospital. I have to keep hold of all the negativity. I have to remember how it stops me going out and playing sport, and keeps me detached from reality. This is no way to live. My anorexia is not going to be a life sentence.

16th July 2008

Grandma's BMI is now 15, so at least she is putting on weight. When I'm her age, I want to be out there having fun with my grandchildren. That sounds like another motivation!

Lizzie said I still looked very thin – that means it was a successful day!

25th July 2008

Today was tough. I got completely stuck at lunchtime, and even with the constant prompts I couldn't go on, and my motivational cards didn't help. I feel like I have been working at fighting Anorexia for so long now. It is so crap how she still brings me down. Why me? Why was this my destiny? Have I failed? Have I let everyone down?

31st July 2008

Katy got discharged today. I felt a pang of jealousy as she left the centre. Was I jealous she was out? Or jealous she could now eat what she wanted without being watched?

1st August 2008

I was allowed out to go and do a mission trip to Romania with the church. It was so much fun. I spent a lot of the first day in a mess, but I tried to copy what the other girls ate so that I had some guidance. Not even calorie-counting expert, Hope Virgo, can tell you what is in this Romanian food!

I lost a couple of kilograms during my time in Romania. Not sure if this is good or bad. No one really notices a tiny bit of weight loss, but to me it seems huge. It also scares me that I don't know how much I should be eating.

30th August 2008

Running along the Portway in Bristol, I thought back over the last year and prayed. Prayer never seems to work, but maybe the fact I had come this far was a miracle in itself. I looked up and saw a rainbow shining in the sky. It was so beautiful, and I felt inspired.

11th September 2008

Not long until I get discharged. Caroline says they wouldn't let me go if they didn't think I could cope, but I still feel so reliant on the unit. I know I want to stay well, I'm just not sure how much energy I have to fight on. At least we had an agreement with the ED unit in Birmingham that they are allowed to contact my parents if my BMI dips under 18. In the last few weeks I have become so conscious of people commenting on my weight. I like it when people say that I look thin.

15th September 2008

Can't believe it is my last day at the unit tomorrow. It is weird leaving an institution where I have lived nearly full-time for the last year. I have sunk into the daily life, and missed all the fun of leaving school, but survived! I can't believe that this time last year, I nearly died. But now I am very much alive, and I have my coping mechanisms for when times get tough. Let's hope I don't get re-admitted ever! This has been the hardest year so far but I can't waste it by getting sick again.

January, 2008

Dear Andy

I thought I would write to you and try to explain a few things so that, first, you don't blame yourself for anything that has happened, and second, it might help you understand a bit more about me.

It isn't you that has made me unwell. Please – even if you get nothing out of this letter, please know that.

There are a number of reasons why anorexia starts, mainly emotional reasons, although some research shows a genetic vulnerability to it, which means some people are more prone to it than others. There may be something specific that triggers it, or a number of cumulative things. The eating disorder is the only way in which someone feels able to express themselves.

I am still not entirely sure what triggered mine off. There have been a number of ideas, some are reasons associated with feeling better about myself and about being thinner, knowing that guys find me less attractive and therefore leave me alone when I'm out. It also means that when someone likes me, I know it is because of me, not what I look like.

I do find it difficult when people get too close and when I have to explain how I feel. Controlling my eating has always been a way to get an easy reward and push all my problems away.

I have got to the stage where I know there is a problem and I want to get better. I know that my anorexia is ruining everything that means anything to me: friends, family, sport, and you. I don't want to live like this anymore, but I find it so hard to make myself eat. When I get told to eat at the right times, I do, but it is not very easy for me. I really wish it was, as it's so frustrating. (I had your chocolates as a snack, four at a time, and they were lovely.) However, these feelings don't go away and sometimes I just give up because it feels like too much effort when I have to cry or talk my way through reasons why I should eat.

You are nothing to do with my eating. Sometimes I think you would like me better if I was thinner, especially because I think that thinner girls are more attractive. But obviously, my perception of myself is a little messy. Logically, my BMI is very low, but I still think I am fatter than some people with a higher BMI.

I can't ask you to understand, because I know it is a weird problem, but I do think everyone has problems that are just as bad as mine, except maybe not as obvious, or as life-threatening. But please, don't let the fact you don't understand affect us.

I hope this starts to explain things. If you have had had enough just say – don't stay with me out of pity.

All my love,

Hope xxx

CHAPTER 11

DISCHARGE FROM HOSPITAL

If I could have sent a letter to my eighteen-year-old self, this is what I would have told her.

Dear Hope,

I know you are absolutely terrified of leaving hospital, but you need to remember everything you have learnt this year. It is scary being left on your own, but you won't ever really be alone. I promise. You have people around you who love and care about you. Even when you shut them out, they won't give up on you, but instead they will try to draw you closer. They will be patient and understanding so you just need to try and open up a little bit more. Try not to box those emotions up. It isn't worth it. Pushing people away is pointless and achieves nothing.

Hang on to everything you have learnt, and hang on to those motivations that keep you well. Looking back at you from where I am now has been eye-opening. I remember hospital as if it was yesterday and as I sit here and reflect back, it's 11.03 on a Sunday and that means it is 300-calorie snack time!

I know you are scared of getting sick, but stick with the fight, girl. You can do it. Life is so much better when it isn't being governed by Anorexia. She really isn't your friend. Whatever she tells you, it is all lies! She doesn't really care like your real friends do.

When you doubt yourself and the purpose of your recovery, remember that it is all worth it. You want a job and you want to help others. You'll get a job and you WILL help others. Don't be ashamed of your anorexia and don't be ashamed of feeling things. I know this is tough but feelings are exciting; they make you who you are. Use everything you have learnt this year to help others.

I hate her for ruining your life. I hate her for ruining so many relationships. And I hate her for making you miss out on so much amazing stuff. Hold on to the good times, and don't let her smack you down. She will try. She will try so hard, and there will be times when you will want to give up. But please don't. Please don't ever give in to her. She is full of false promises. She is a fake best friend who does not give a shit about you or how you feel. Please, I beg you to just hang in there.

Love, Hope (aged twenty-six)

I had dreamt of this day for so long and I couldn't quite believe it was finally here. I didn't know if I was scared or excited, but I knew I couldn't spend my entire life in hospital.

My life would be my own again. I couldn't wait to get up when I wanted, to be able to go for a run when I wanted. I already knew exactly where I was going to run. Turn left out of the house, run down the hill and head into the woods. I could almost smell the wood-scented air and feel the mud splatter up my legs.

When it happened, getting discharged was terrifying. While I had been spending less time in the hospital, I was still scared about not having someone to check in with. When I had first gone into hospital, I had dreamt of this day as a way to relapse. I had been planning to get my weight back down as quickly as possible and befriend Anorexia again. I had promised her so many times that I would let her back in. But now I was in a different place. I had discovered what a nasty, manipulative, control freak she really was, and I didn't know if I wanted her back.

My mind wandered to the calories I could cut out and the weight I could lose. Think of the running I could do with no one monitoring me.

But was that what I really wanted?

It had been a tough year, but deep down, I knew I wanted to stay well. I wanted to go to university and experience life again. I had always been very career driven and I wanted to make a difference in the world. None of that would be possible if I was sick. And I hoped that the fear of getting unwell would motivate me to keep fighting, every single day.

The final few sessions I'd had at the hospital were all about preparing me for discharge, but there had still been times when I felt I wasn't strong enough. One snack time, Laura had a chocolate bar with only 210 calories – a whole ninety calories less than we were supposed to have – and I was furious. Somehow, she had been allowed to eat it. It was ridiculous how it had made me so cross, and that made me think I just wasn't ready to leave. Supposing I started judging what others were eating around me? How would that impact me and affect my recovery?

I sat on a bench outside the hospital with Simon, one of the nurses that I'd always really liked, and he helped me realise I was just scared. And I hoped that the fact I was so scared about managing on my own meant I probably did want to make it.

At 4 pm they brought out a cake for me. The day before, they'd asked me what sort of cake I liked. I didn't even know if I liked cake. No! That was something I still couldn't face eating. I checked the calories and then felt the guilt. Was I really ready to leave? How was I going to cope at university?

I was ready to chicken out. I didn't know if I could actually do this. I had been so unwell, and my anorexia had done nothing for me, but I almost felt I could hear her reassuring me, saying, 'Come on, Hope, pull yourself together. You want this. You want your life back. You want to go to university and you want to travel, and you can't do any of it you stay unwell.' The words rang through me and this time, she was right.

I knew that a year ago, I would have gone straight back to my old ways. Even six months earlier, I wouldn't have been able to stay well, but I felt like I had enough resolve now. It was time to jump in at the deep end and try.

I looked around the room at the girls and boys who I had spent so much time with. So many of them were still struggling, still "masked up". I knew I would miss them (well, most of them). I was allowed to stay in touch with people, but inevitably I was encouraged to only spend time with people who were doing well. That wiped out half the room straightaway.

I still didn't trust some of the other girls and their anorexia. I didn't trust that they would try hard to stay well. I kept in touch with Katy and saw her a few times in the first year after I was discharged. It was nice seeing her, knowing she was doing okay. But was she really? On Facebook she always looked happy. But when we met up, it felt like we were never 100% confident with our eating. After that initial year, we said we'd meet again, but we never did. I guess we just couldn't face the prospect of delving into our past again.

So that was how I left. I thanked the staff, and then, without a backwards glance, I headed off home. I thought I would never, ever, step foot in that hospital again. (Since leaving, I have been back a couple of times: once for a session with my psychologist after my first term at university, and once for a catch-up coffee before I went travelling.)

That evening, I got back home and had dinner with my family. Mum did Quorn sausages and a jacket potato for me. I felt everyone watching me as I ate, and tears started to well up in my eyes. Was I really ready for this? What if it all went wrong? And what if I never felt okay again?

I spent the evening sorting through my hospital stuff. I created a box of things to help me stay well (it still sits under my bed in my flat in London). I read through the messages in my goodbye card and they all rang true: I was a fighter, they said. I was determined. And I had survived this far – I had to keep going now. They believed in me; I just needed the confidence to believe in myself.

It felt strange to be back in my room. The smell of vomit still seemed to hang in the air. The stains were indelibly printed on the carpet. Everything was exactly how I had left it. It was still my room and I still felt the same need to be alone there.

The next evening was less strained. Everyone chatted for ages. But as I finished my meal, I started to get agitated. I wanted to leave the table. I just didn't get it – yes, eating was sociable but I was ready to move to the next room. I sat there restlessly, my mind wandering again.

I still felt uneasy. I asked my older sister to come and sit on the floor while I showered. I didn't want the temptation to make myself sick. At 8 pm, Dad knocked on my bedroom door and told me it was time for my snack. 300 calories, no more, no less. I knew he was trying to help, but it was just so annoying. Would my family ever be able to relax around me? Or would Anorexia hang over us forever now?

After being at home a few days, I was already worried about my weight. On the Sunday, Mum took me to buy some good scales so I could manage my weight when I was at university. The rule was that I was allowed to weigh myself once a week. But only once.

My family was doing everything they could to help me settle back in, but it was still easier to be emotionally unengaged. For that first week, we stuck to regimented dinner times. I would come down to the kitchen about 5.30 pm to make sure my food was being prepared with no extra bits. If dinner wasn't ready to eat at 6 pm on the dot, I would start to get agitated. Looking back, it must have been so annoying for everyone, but at the time, I didn't care.

One of the hardest evenings was when James wanted to go to an all-you-can-eat restaurant for his birthday. I didn't get the point of those restaurants at all. Mum told me that she'd help me choose what to have, but it still stressed me out, knowing we would be there for hours with so much food around.

For the best part of a year, I had been weighing out pasta and eating out of yoghurt pots! Now, I was faced with mountains of food. In the middle of the table, there was a chocolate fountain. I loved chocolate, but I knew I wouldn't let myself have any.

I looked around. Where the hell would I start? I felt myself heating up, the sweat seeping through my clothes. I just wanted to get out of there. I felt Mum's hand grabbing mine and her words in my ear, 'We can do this, Hope!'

Mum and Kate were brilliant. They helped guide me through it, and somehow, I made it. I didn't particularly enjoy it – and I spent most of the evening frantically adding up the calories on my plate and everyone else's, but I had done it.

Dear Mollie,

I am sorry for putting you through what I did. I know it can't have been easy for you growing up and having to visit me in hospital. You were so young, you shouldn't have had to go through that. I look at you now and I do worry that my mental health impacted you. I worry that I changed how you think about food and body image, and I am so sorry if that is the case.

You mean the world to me and the last thing I want is to have ever hurt you.

I love you my baby sister. xxx

Dear Samuel,

I am sorry that you had to watch me killing myself slowly. I am sorry for the day that you had to watch me eat my breakfast as instructed by Mum, and then throw the food into a plant pot. When I think back, it's quite funny to imagine I would ever have got away with that.

I am sorry that you felt you had failed Mum when I hadn't eaten and disappeared out the house. I am sorry that I was so difficult to be around and that you had to deal with it while you had so much other stuff going on.

My anorexia turned me into a selfish person and I am definitely not proud of the way I behaved. When I look back at it, whether in terms of my feelings, or in a more matter-of-fact way, I feel embarrassed and upset that my actions hurt you so much.

Thank you for not giving up on me and for being there when I came out of hospital.

I love you Samey. x

Hope's mum:

Hope's return from hospital was very gradual over the summer of 2008. The plan was for her to be fully discharged from hospital in September, ready for university, so she still spent a huge amount of the summer at the hospital. The times when she went back to hospital gave me a bit of respite, just some time to switch off from the reality of the situation. That summer I saw some glimpses of the old Hope and I longed for her to be back. We joked about food occasionally and we had some open and frank conversations about how she was feeling. But after the conversation, she would snap back, shut down and switch off.

One of my most vivid memories was when we went on a holiday to Munich in July. Hope didn't want to come and was still under the supervision of the hospital with her eating. It was so relaxing not having to maintain the rigid mealtimes that had become such a feature of our family life. The holiday was a welcome relief, and as soon as I realised that, I felt guilty. Did it mean I was a bad mother because I was thinking in this way?

At the airport, waiting for the return flight, Hope's youngest brother suddenly started to sob silently. This was so out of character for Samuel. He was quiet most of the time, and hid his emotions well. Even during family therapy, he had managed to keep things close. I looked at him, my heart hurting, and asked, 'What's the matter?'

His reply was short and sharp. 'I don't want to go back to all that!'

I knew the last year had been a strain on everyone but in that moment, I saw that it had been a completely shit year for everyone. In the absence of three elder siblings, Samuel had essentially been catapulted into a position of responsibility in the family, and it was hard for him. I thought back to when Samuel told me that Hope had said she'd eaten her toast before school, when really, she'd hidden it in a plant pot. He had felt so responsible for her. And a week later she had gone into hospital. I had reassured him at the time, telling him it wasn't his fault, but my words were full of emptiness. By that point I had run out of energy.

I think it's easy to forget what a strain mental illness is on other members of the family, especially brothers and sisters. Mealtimes were very difficult – about an hour prior to meals, Hope needed to see me preparing the food. She would hover in the kitchen (to check I didn't sneak anything extra into the food). The pressure of having to prepare a meal under her watchful eye was intense, and I often found myself buckling under the pressure. I knew I wasn't supposed to show the pressure, and that just made it feel even worse.

Life was tough, and I very rarely felt like I had done what was best for everybody. For me it was a time of trying to do my best, but frequently falling short.

It was a different sort of worry when Hope went to university in September, but things gradually seemed to return to normal ...

CHAPTER 12

GOING TO UNIVERSITY

Hope's mum:
Hope was off to university – she had made it!

I had been up to the campus with her and we'd done the trial meals so that she knew exactly what she needed to buy and eat for each meal. I was so immensely proud of the fact that she "made it" and continued to manage her recovery with very little direct intervention.

We just had to trust that Hope could do it. That was hard. But I had faith in her.

Hope:
I flung myself into getting ready for university. I ran lots, but tried to stick to the hospital routine. There was a never-ending battle raging in my head. Following a year of hospital life with strict bed times, mealtimes and snack times, I worried that I might have become institutionalised. Was I now going to carry those ingrained habits with me wherever I went?

I hoped that getting away from home, and all the memories of my anorexia, would help make things better. Well, that was the plan, although it still meant my life wasn't very flexible. I'd panic if it got to 6.15 pm and we hadn't begun dinner, and I would stress about fitting all my calories in. That target of 2,500 calories seemed like a mountain each day.

I had thought that by the time I left hospital, I would be completely fine. That I wouldn't have to weigh myself, and I could eat whatever I wanted without feeling fat. But when I left, I knew I wasn't better. I lived in fear of failing. I was still so confused about food. Perhaps if I took each day as it came, things would get better? It was hard work managing it like that, but I knew that if I tried to look any further ahead, it would just freak me out.

Before I left, Mum stocked up the fridge with foods I would like and some easy meals to get me started. She'd sit with me while I struggled my way through them, bite by bite. I tried to put on a brave face, but inside I was breaking apart. The battle with Anorexia was entering a new phase. I didn't know if I should listen to her. I knew she'd let me down, but how could I push her out of my life when she had been such a vital part of me, and such a trusted friend for so long?

In that last week, I tried to pick up where I'd left off with my friends. But it was hard to fit back in. Even though they had come to visit me a lot throughout the year, and I'd been on occasional nights out with them over the summer, I didn't really know how to act around them. People would ask where I'd been after my exams (they'd all been away to Zante) so I didn't exactly want to say I'd been stuck in a mental health hospital!

I couldn't shake the feeling that people were watching me. I still feel that same sensation at times now. As soon as people find out about my anorexia, I can feel them looking me up and down. I can see them watching what I eat. I can almost hear them thinking I can't possibly be anorexic – because I don't look it.

I was very well aware of my triggers – the little things that set me off – but during my time in hospital I had developed coping mechanisms to help me. It was all about taking one day at a time and making sure I didn't slip into bad habits that would be hard to break. My mechanisms were simple:

1. Stick to 2,500 calories a day
2. Have at least one day off from exercise a week
3. Eat three meals and three snacks every day

4. Remember that my feelings around food are in my head and are not my reality
5. Remember my motivations
6. Remember how Anorexia ruined my life

My coping mechanisms empowered me and guided me through the days after my discharge. They helped. But I was still afraid that the battle would never end, that I would never, ever feel thin. In a way, I think that living with the fear was a good thing. And using my regimented structure to help me face the fear kept me well.

Mum drove me to university on the Sunday and we talked openly in the car. I was on edge, wondering how I would stick to my eating plan. I admitted that I was scared and didn't know how I was going to stay well. She assured me I would. She had faith in me, and I knew I had to prove to everyone that I could manage this. I wanted to make them proud.

On my first night, everyone was given two drinks tokens. I gave one to my new friend, Emily, as I hadn't drunk properly for ages. I didn't think I could handle my drink any more. (She still laughs about how much of a lightweight I was). We had a barbecue and headed to the student bar down the road. I don't remember eating much. I had no idea where to start with a barbecue. What would I eat? Would I have too much, too little? What size would the portions be? My way of compensating was to drink. I knew how many calories were in every bit of alcohol and knew the portions would be okay for me to manage.

Was this what my university life was going to be like? Not eating, but simply coping by drinking too much?

CHAPTER 13

I SURVIVED 365 DAYS OUT OF HOSPITAL

Early into my first term, I got drunk and opened up to Emily about my anorexia. She was so supportive. It didn't even matter that she didn't really understand; it was just nice telling someone. She didn't question the fact that I had to have dinner at 6 pm each night and I had this hospital bowl to eat my cereal out of because I then knew exactly how many bran flakes to put in the bowl.

Not everyone was so understanding though. The medical centre gave me Prozac. In my diary, I wrote:

I am not depressed. Fact. Loads of people feel shit the whole time. Fact. They just want to stop me coming to the sessions. Fact. Prozac saves them time. Fact!

Even though I still felt unsure of who I really was and what I looked like, my first term flew by. I was coping. Instead of getting preoccupied with challenging different food groups, I stuck rigidly to my eating plan. I knew when I hadn't had enough and I found that I was in a good enough position to be able to correct myself. Otherwise, I'd drink alcohol to make up the calories.

The days merged into each other as I got up stupidly early to exercise, did my work, and then started on the drinking again. I knew that I wasn't dependent on the alcohol, but I still felt so insecure about what I looked like and what people thought of me, that my confidence was easily crushed. So I resorted to drinking to get my confidence back.

I had been warned about slipping back into old habits, and after struggling for a couple of weeks in that first term, I pulled myself out of the hole. I knew I had to, or else drop out. But I was also determined to show everyone that I could stay well without antidepressants. If I started to show any signs of being unwell again, I knew Mum and Dad would interfere – and I definitely didn't want to go home. Sure enough, Mum said I looked a bit thin when I got back from my first term. I knew I was going to have to watch her very carefully so she didn't make me eat more than I should.

So I pulled myself up, gritted my teeth, and fought on. I was still sticking to my eating plan, but weighing myself most days to help keep the stress at bay. It helped me feel like I was getting some of the control back.

My first Christmas since leaving hospital was strange! I still felt like I was being watched. The day went well, everyone seemed to be getting along, and I had some great presents. But I was aware that I had become even better at wearing a mask to hide the tears I was trying to fight off.

Kate got married during the holidays and I survived the hen party and the wedding. Her wedding had been another one of those targets – a date in the diary when I thought I'd be cured of Anorexia. But I was disappointed. I remember Mum saying that I looked thinner again, but she was probably just trying to trick me. It always confused me when people said things like this. Part of me was so happy, but the other part of me just assumed they were tricking me, that they wanted me to start "letting go" of that control. Maybe that would justify giving me more food in her mind, which completely panicked me.

In the new year, I realised that the hospital hadn't been in contact with me again, and I began to wonder if they thought I was too fat to be diagnosed with Anorexia any more. I wondered if it would make a difference if I suddenly lost a lot of weight. But a week or so later, they rang to make an appointment. I couldn't say if things were getting better or worse. I still had days when I weighed out my cereal, and days when I calorie counted every single portion, but they were getting less frequent and I wasn't being as strict with myself as I had been. I knew I needed to let go and experiment with my food more; I just wasn't ready yet. I wasn't sure if I would ever be ready.

Fat days still came around a couple of times a week. Sometimes they were easy to deal with, sometimes they weren't. One day in February, I was in my room when the feelings swamped me. I felt worthless and huge. I wasn't really sure what to do. Trying to fight off the need to go for another run, I emailed Dad hoping for some insightful thoughts. Instead, I got an email back saying, 'I am sure the feeling will pass.' How could he say that?! Maybe they'd always thought that way, right through my recovery. It was as if he was returning to a passive state, coping by focusing on his work. But I was furious. It seemed like such an uncaring response.

I wondered what I would have wanted Dad to say. If he had said I was fat, I would lose weight. If he had said I was thin, I doubt I would have believed it, and would have dismissed it as a sympathetic ideal. It frustrated me that there wasn't a simple solution to all of this – something to say that could undo all the confusion and take away the pain.

Later, I got a message from Dad apologising for sounding so dismissive, but it was already too late. I went for a run, uncertain about how much I could turn to him any more.

As term two moved on, I found myself getting more caught up in my own world. I still lacked the confidence to try different things, but I wanted to stay well so much now. And I didn't mind eating the same foods each day as long as my weight stayed up. So I returned to the same diet of calorie-counted sandwiches.

Just wanting to stay well was never enough. It was so hard. I cried endlessly about my eating. I would sit in my room and wonder what had gone wrong and where I would be if I hadn't got help. I started looking over my old review letters, and when I felt really bad, Mum would remind me of just how much worse it had been when I was ill.

I found it difficult being around the boys at university when they were loud, and I was gradually losing confidence in my dress sense. I started choosing bigger jumpers more often. I wasn't enjoying this emotional rollercoaster and I felt stuck. It all seemed so stupid; I didn't even have anything to show I was ill any more.

But then, something changed. Maybe it was because I'd had such a "fat" week. My eating and my weight seemed to be all over the place. I arrived at the hospital expecting it to be the same as ever, but for once, I genuinely felt able to open up, although I still wasn't able to let myself cry publicly, even when the tears welled up in my eyes.

I was reminded that people do get better from eating disorders: about 40% of people who have had an eating disorder never think about it again. Amazingly only 15% of people are unable to fight it off and stay stuck with their disorder. The rest can continue to live with it, supported by their coping mechanisms. I wondered which category I would fall into. But at that point in my life, the prospect of not thinking about it – or not feeling compelled to exercise – seemed so far off. I was encouraged to stick to simple steps.

By now I knew the signs of slipping back into this cycle, such as weighing myself more than once a day, running more and counting calories more often. I needed to challenge these things if I really wanted to stay on top of my recovery. It would be stupid now to give it all up.

But other times, it frustrated me that I would still manage to eat, even when I felt so low. Anorexia was such a potent, visible sign of dissatisfaction that, by comparison, eating just looked like giving in. It certainly didn't do anything to show the turmoil I was feeling inside.

Back at the hospital in May, I was beginning to learn that so many of my thoughts were irrational, but that was annoying because I didn't know why I still felt them. I had to draw a pie chart summing up my life; half of the pie was devoted to my weight, and the other bits were sport, friends and going out. I wished that the weight thing wasn't such a big part of the chart, but it was an honest assessment. I wondered what made up other people's charts ...

By the time my first year at university was drawing to a close, I thought about how I had managed to maintain my recovery. I was so pleased that I had been able to stay well for so long without slipping too far back into my old ways. Of course, I still had irrational days, but they were becoming easier to cope with and much less frequent. The downside was that when I did have a bad day, it threw me so much. Then the following day, I'd realise just how irrational I'd been.

I still calorie counted, and I knew I had to let this go too. I didn't know what was stopping me, but I just didn't feel ready yet. I imagined what it would feel like to get up in the morning without feeling fat, and without a compulsion to exercise or count calories. In a way, these things were all a part of my identity now. And I wondered if I could ever re-write my personality in such a dramatic way. Something would have to change first.

I'd heard that people with anorexia had been able to let it go when something had "clicked" for them. It had happened to Susan; but I didn't know what needed to click for me. Emily told me she thought that things were clicking, but she didn't know how much I was weighing myself, how much I was exercising, and that I was still counting my calories. I hoped and hoped that maybe the next summer I would feel something "click". What I wanted was an overnight fix, but I wasn't sure how I was going to go about finding it. Maybe for some people it was a more long-term thing; I just knew that I didn't want to be in that percentage of people who stayed struggling, unhappy and ill. What sort of life would that be?

The hospital encouraged me to challenge my food more, count calories less, and be more willing to try different things. I wish I could, but it seemed so scary. On the day of the summer ball, I fixated on my worries about the food. It was odd thinking that everyone else would just turn up without thinking about it, and I really wished I could be in that group of people.

I had bought a nice dress, but when I tried it on and looked in the mirror the day before the ball, I felt like a purple berry. I hated it, and burst into tears. I immediately began to slip back into thinking about when I could skip snacks and meals without people realising. I was confused; the dress had fitted when I bought it, and I hadn't let myself put on any weight, so I didn't know what the reality was.

I stuffed it back into the bag and went to bed. I couldn't find an explanation for what was wrong with the dress. Looking back, I was glad that I managed to move past it, but I still think I looked fat at the ball. I compared myself to every other person in the room and felt huge compared to all of them. Even though I knew that was completely irrational thinking, it didn't help me feel any better.

I'd made it through the first year at university and even though it still felt scary, I was getting better at pushing myself my boundaries. I was becoming more and more determined to crack this. I wasn't going to let Anorexia rule my life.

But life kept pushing back ...

I spent a month interrailing around Europe in the summer and I knew I could handle it if I just ate what Katie ate over the month. The night before I was due to go, Mum took me out for a coffee. I thought that she just wanted to double check that I was sorted for the trip, but no. It was to tell me that she and Dad had decided to get divorced.

I was livid. Anorexia had kept them together for another year, but no longer. James once told me that he thought something terrible needed to happen to bring our parents back together, and I thought that my nearly dying would have done that. But perhaps the stress had actually pushed them further away from each other.

I headed off the next morning, still cross with my parents. I had so many questions, but once again, I pretended I was fine. Thank God I was going away for a month, so I could try to forget about it all. The food was okay, and I managed quite well. It was a brilliant month and I felt happy. I only ran twice over the whole month, which for me was a huge achievement. And while I was excited to return to running when I got home, I enjoyed my time away. Katie and Helen were so supportive the whole time and I was so grateful for them. When Dad picked us up when we got back, he commented on how thin I looked. I felt a warm feeling inside, happy that I had lost weight while being away. How ridiculous was I?

CHAPTER 14

LIVING A DOUBLE LIFE

At this stage I was finally feeling like I was starting to enjoy life. The first year of university had been brilliant. I'd stayed well, and although I'd still exercised a lot and counted the calories in everything, I felt like I'd turned things around. Food wasn't a dirty word any more. I had even begun to enjoy unexpected pub dinners and last-minute cooking and drinking sessions with my housemates. My friends helped make me happy. For the first time in God knows how long, I started to wonder if maybe, just maybe, I was ready to let my anorexia go.

But when you have had a mental health problem, it's hard to know if you are ever completely over it, or if it will always be there under the surface, waiting to take control. Anorexia was like an ex. No matter how far I moved on, there was still that temptation to stay in touch. There were times when I'd catch myself thinking about her, or wondering about what would happen if I let her back into my life. And I knew she was only ever one or two bad days away.

I was starting to feel the pressure to have that "perfect" university life. There was always that sense of having to go out and have fun. Maybe I was trying to prove to myself that I could be that happy-go-lucky person – the "normal" girl with "normal" thoughts.

To help me relax, I decided to join a running club. I didn't do it to please her, but looking back, it was the catalyst Anorexia needed to come back ...

Competition at the club was high, especially as it was dominated by men. I felt the pressure, but I thrived on it. It was exhilarating to be racing again. Tearing round the track – 400 metres steady, 400 metres sprinting – I absolutely loved it. And I was good. I felt valued in the club and I wanted to please everyone. Most of all, I wanted to impress the coach, so I began to train more and push myself further.

There were days when I would go out for a run twice a day. I knew it was silly, and I could feel the old obsessions creeping back, but I couldn't help myself. The contentment, the thrill, and the feeling of being good at something was so important to me. I felt like I was in complete control of what I was doing. I thought I could handle Anorexia, so I buried her voice as deep as I could and carried on.

But how do you go on resisting temptation, day after day?

As my running increased, I could feel my body shutting down again. I knew I was slipping back into bad habits, and I hated myself for it.

I pretended I was fine. It was the easy thing to do. But I knew I was in real danger of slipping under her control and wasting everything I'd learnt in hospital. Those thoughts kept nagging away at me under the surface. I rationalised it all with myself, saying it was okay to keep exercising this much because I was eating well. I tried bargaining with myself too – thinking that if I kept count of all my calories, I'd be able to retain control. But I was slipping fast, pushing myself harder and harder, trying to disguise any pain and doubt with exercise.

I knew I had to admit it to myself – to acknowledge that I was over-training, but I kept putting it off. I wasn't ready to face my worries head on, not yet. And so, in the meantime, I continued to go running. I thought that as long as I ate enough, I'd get away with it. But I also knew that I didn't want to live my life dictated by exercise. I didn't want to feel guilty every time I felt I hadn't done enough. And I knew that something was going to give eventually.

I started to feel pain in my right foot whenever I ran. I knew my bones were weak from being unwell for so long. It was scary, but I told myself that it was all in my head. It had to be. I was still able to run, so I just kept on running through the pain, dosing up on painkillers morning and night. I iced my foot after running, and slept with it raised. But steadily the pain got worse until, one evening, it was absolutely unbearable.

I hobbled home across the downs from my shift at work, and I knew had no choice but to go to the hospital for an x-ray.

I sat there fidgeting in the waiting room while I waited for the results. My foot was throbbing and I felt on edge. I was angry at everyone. And I was scared, not just because of my foot, but because I could hear that familiar voice whispering in my ear again. I knew I had let Anorexia down by coming here. I should have been able to push through the pain.

Finally, I got the results: the metatarsals in my foot had snapped.

Fear flooded through me. How was I going to be able to exercise now?

I limped out of the hospital on my crutches, got into the car next to James and sat in silence. I was terrified.

Terrified of living with Anorexia. Terrified of living without her.

Terrified of the weight gain. How would I be able to go on eating without the exercise to take off the calories? What would I do when I had a bad day? I relied on running so much to kick-start my mood on bad days. How would I cope without it? I couldn't see a way through the turmoil I was feeling.

Anorexia started shouting at me.

'You're going to get fat again!'

'You need to stop eating!'

'You need to find ways to exercise!'

'If you let this affect your weight, or if you let this stop your exercise, you'll be a total failure. You'll be no good for anything. No good for anyone.'

Maybe she was right. Maybe I was a failure.

I felt so guilty for letting her down. I got home and put on a brave face and I said I was fine. I kept on saying it, whenever anyone asked. I don't even know how many times I lied about the way I really felt; I lost track after the first few times. It was always easier to lie about how I was feeling. And the more I said it, the easier it was to take a bit more control over my food. I started finding sneaky ways to work out too.

Part of me knew I had to admit how I felt to someone. I had to tell someone I was struggling, but I felt so lost and helpless. And so I kept it all under wraps. I smiled, popped on my mask every morning, and instead of talking, I let the guilt build up inside me. I managed to squeeze in gym sessions on the exercise bike or the cross trainer, and I was so proud of myself for finding a way around my injury. I knew Anorexia was proud of me too. But at the same time I kept thinking to myself, *Why am I slipping? Why is she guilt-tripping me? Why am I so lost in this?'*

I carried on like this for weeks, hiding my true feelings away in the day, and going out more in the evenings to try and "anaesthetise" myself. Somehow, I managed to pretend I was fine for the entire Christmas holidays! Maybe I wasn't such a failure after all.

By the time I made my way back up to Birmingham, the snow was settling. It made the crutches even more of a nightmare, and I knew it was going to be even harder to get out and exercise. The gym was a good ten-minute run away, and with crutches in the snow, God knows how long it would take. But I was determined, and one snowy day I managed it. I half walked, half limped through snow, on crutches. To go to the gym! I was so proud of myself, elated even. But then, reality hit me – I had a broken metatarsal. What the hell was I doing going to the gym? It was ridiculous. I knew I was heading back to a "double life". What I let people see on the surface didn't have anything to do with what was going on inside.

I knew I had to act quickly if I was going to stop Anorexia taking her hold on me again. I could feel her close by, ready to pounce.

Letting her back in was not worth it. I knew I had to stay strong. Part of me actually felt lucky she was back, reassuring me she was a stable part of my life. But at the same time, she made me question my first year at university.

I'd had such a good first year, but now, thanks to her, I was starting to think that had been the exception. That hadn't been real. This was real. This is what my life had been like for years. I had presented a picture of security and togetherness to the world, but gone on struggling inside. Perhaps I was lucky that my anorexia had broken me and hospitalised me a few years before. That's what had forced me to face the reality of my double life. I didn't know what true happiness was any more. How can you be truly happy when you've got so used to pretending to be happy?

I knew I wasn't the only one. I was sure many people lived double lives without anyone else ever knowing – perhaps as a way to protect the people around them, to stop them worrying by pretending that everything was okay. It scared me to think of how many people I knew who were hiding their true feelings like this, living their lives in silence. I thought about my friendship group. I thought about how we all spent so much time talking, without ever really saying anything. We were young and we were having a good time. What did any of us have to be sad, scared or miserable about? Is that how we thought? Is that how everyone thinks?

We were all so eager to try to prove what an amazing time we were having, all of the time. I used to hate it if I tried to talk to someone and they'd bat all my questions away if they thought I was getting too close to talking about their feelings. But now I knew I was turning into one of those people too; I was only thinking in terms of calories and exercise. My own feelings didn't matter.

But I knew I desperately didn't want to live that way again, and I didn't want people around me to have to live like that either. And so I decided to try being more open about my feelings, so that at least others might feel like they were able to talk about theirs, and maybe I could help myself a bit in the process.

I was lucky to have such a tight group of friends. Emily and Nikki were amazing. They stuck by me and stayed patient when I had a bad day. I wasn't asking anyone else to try to understand; I didn't even know how to explain what was going on with me, and I didn't want people to think I was weird. But I knew having them there, and being able to share my feelings with them, really helped me.

Since leaving hospital, this was the first challenge I had come up against that really pushed my resolve. Now that I was getting to the point where I finally felt able to talk about how I was feeling, instead of channelling all my pain into my anorexia, I had to make sure I managed my eating and exercise. I thought back to what had helped me in hospital. I knew that exercise was one of my triggers and I read back over information on exercise and food. I looked back through my hospital diary and tried to remind myself that I had achieved nothing by being anorexic. Instead, I had nearly died.

I wrote down what had helped me before, and I thought about my motivations for staying healthy – and that started to help me more and more. I was tired of fighting Anorexia and at times I would go back to my hospital routine. Sometimes I relied on my mum to message me to check I was eating. I knew deep down that, having done it once, I had the power to beat Anorexia again, before she ruined my life.

I wasn't going to let her destroy me. All I wanted and needed was a normal life at university, without her dictating my every move. I deserved that. I was lucky to have such a tight-knit group of friends around me, and a family who cared so deeply for me. I realised that I would never underestimate the power of talking to them all. I found it hard at first, but the more I did it, the easier it got. I didn't really want them to check up on me, but simply telling them I was struggling made things easier. It helped take away my guilt when I wasn't exercising. It helped me shake off Anorexia's grip – for a while, at least.

I knew then my old friend had always been close by, trying to worm her way back in, and I didn't feel like I had beaten her yet, but I had a group of friends who were so much better, kinder, and more supportive than she ever was. Emily and Nikki will have no idea how much they helped me throughout my university life.

The three years at university presented a range of challenges, from big things like breaking my foot, to little things like eating out at mealtimes. When I left hospital, they told me I would either survive or get sick again. I was too determined and too stubborn to give in. I was going to prove the doubters wrong; I was going to show them I could stay well.

For me, being away from a family home where there were so many unhappy memories helped. It wasn't that I'd had an unpleasant childhood, but the secrecy, the lies, and the guilt of the last few years were a constant reminder of what I had been through. Just like the stains on my carpet.

I wanted to let all the bad memories go now, and begin to feel like I was living a normal life. I knew that being at university had helped me stay well. There had been tough times, but I had kept going. Emily, who lived with me for the whole three years, could see a change in me from day one. She loved how much more relaxed I was around food.

I remember one summer's evening when Nikki, Emily and I sat on the Southbank, sharing a bottle of wine. We were sitting there soaking up the sun, with sweat trickling down our backs, when out of the blue, Emily said, 'I can't believe how far you've come.' We thought back to what I'd been like at the beginning, laughed about my silly bowl for an exact amount of cereal, and how I'd reacted the day the bowl got smashed. I was even able to laugh at how agitated I'd get if we ate a tiny bit late.

I did still have my ups and downs. There were still days when I woke up feeling huge. So while I was convincing some people that Anorexia had gone, I had come to accept that she was always going to be there. I was frustrated that there were still days when I struggled to function; at times it felt like I was turning into a dysfunctional adult with a mental health problem.

So whenever I felt especially low, I surrounded myself with people. That was easy at university. I loved socialising, and talking to so many different people helped me to keep my thoughts at bay. I knew that whenever I needed them, I could rely on my friends to help me switch off from Anorexia.

Just being at university made me determined to stay well. It showed me what life could be like without Anorexia as my friend. It was obvious to me now that she wasn't the friend I thought she was. I still had to work on accepting that my friends liked me for who I really was, not for who Anorexia had tried to make me.

CHAPTER 15

MY GRANDMA – THE ANOREXIC

My final year at university flew by. Mood-wise, it was fairly mixed, but I coped. In the final few weeks after exams, we went out a lot and drank plenty, but I loved every second with my friends. We spent most nights drinking and sitting up for hours. But I can assure you, I always got my morning exercise in, no matter how hungover I was!

My friend Alicia and I would often get up early on Sunday mornings to run around Selly Park, with fake tan still dribbling down our legs. Sometimes we'd do our normal four-mile loop past Cadbury World, where we could smell the chocolate cooking. To celebrate the end of university, we'd planned to go camping – complete with full-length mirrors – but just as we were getting ready to go, I got a call from Dad saying my grandma had gone back into hospital. She had stopped eating and had completely given up on life. The tell-tale signs of anorexia were eerily familiar ...

I never knew for sure that Grandma struggled with eating, but I remembered Mum once saying she'd often cook a huge lunch for us, but not eat anything herself. And I must have suspected something when I was at my pre-assessment at the hospital; they had asked about any family history of mental health issues and Mum had mentioned her.

I used to love going round to her house when we were growing up, and I was completely oblivious to any signs of anorexia then. We used to go for lunch and then go and look around the local garden centre with Grandad, watching the huge fish swimming in their tanks. We'd then go back for ginger beer and curl up to watch television.

Grandad had died when I was in junior school and Grandma had struggled on without him, distancing herself more and more from the rest of us. Living alone in a huge house must have been tough for her. And I suppose she had already begun to give up on life.

I guess Anorexia held her close, like she did me, on those cold nights when she was alone. It guided her through the grieving process and made her feel whole again. I wish I had known earlier. Maybe I could have intervened, made her feel alive, held her when she wanted to give up on life.

After Dad called, I headed home for the night to say my goodbyes. I didn't know what to expect. I was scared but I knew I'd regret not seeing her one final time. As I walked up to the bed and saw the lady lying there, I thought she didn't look like herself at all. She was tiny. I thought back to the letters I'd written, urging her to eat and get well. She looked awful and I didn't know what I could do to make her feel any different. But as I looked on, I flashed forward in my mind to an image of me as an old lady. The thought that Anorexia could control my entire life hit me hard. I knew I couldn't end my life like that, and I knew I had to stay well.

CHAPTER 16

THRIVING

Negative thoughts are my belief and not my reality.

You are worth more than this so-called anorexia. It will not get you anywhere in life so don't stop fighting it.

I graduated from university in 2011. I had beaten the odds. In many ways, surviving with limited support was even more of an achievement than graduating. I was so pleased that I'd hung in there, and slightly shocked that I'd actually made it.

Mum and Dad had finally divorced, and I actually moved in with Dad and his new wife during the summer. I was angry with my mum. I think I blamed her for the divorce and I was just fed up of her. There had been lots of ups and downs throughout our relationship, but after she'd failed to turn up and watch me take part in the London Marathon earlier that year, I didn't want anything to do with her. I guess the emotion of sorting out our differences was still too much for me, and I wanted to hurt her like she had hurt me. All the distress – the pain, the anger, the sadness – she had caused was buried deep inside me. But it was just too distressing to talk about and too hard to resolve, so I didn't see the point in trying.

James had a girlfriend at the time who also struggled with food. Mum didn't seem to understand how tough that was for me. I used to watch her at mealtimes and secretly wrap my fingers around my wrists and thighs to measure myself in comparison to her. It felt like no one cared. Perhaps because Mum and James had been unable to "fix" me, they had decided their new mission in life was to fix Hazel.

So, typical me, I ran away as soon as the swell of emotions got too much.

Moving in with Dad was fine. He was often at work all day or away on holiday, so he wasn't around a huge amount. And no one ever came up to the top floor where I slept. Their house was lovely and modern, but I never quite felt at home there.

My food got a bit funny that summer; I was out of a routine and out on my own a lot more. Some days I would just forget to eat, and I worried about the food that Dad's new wife would cook. She didn't really understand my eating habits and I couldn't be bothered to explain it to her. I didn't even see the point. There are times when I'm still like that – people don't understand that there are times when it all flares up and makes my life very, very difficult.

My first Saturday night at Dad's, I came back late from St Pauls Carnival. I had tried to shut the front door as quietly as possibly, but failed. The slam of the door shook through the house, and I stood awkwardly in the hallway before creeping up to my bedroom. I missed coming home and seeing that a light had been left on for me, that sense that someone cared where I was. But those uncertain feelings only ever came to me at night. When they did, I would sit with them for a few seconds and then let them go.

Occasionally, Dad and I would go running together. I was much better than him (obviously!) but I enjoyed making him come out with me. It seemed like the only thing I could do on my own with him, without his wife being there.

One thing that has stuck with me forever is a question I asked him while we were out running, and to this day, I don't know why I even asked it. Maybe I just wanted a reason to self-destruct, or find another way to hurt myself. So I asked him whether he would choose me over his new wife or not. He answered awkwardly, but I got the gist. And it hurt.

So, what does Hope Virgo do? What did I do when my mum pissed me off? I ran! I got the first job I could in London and left.

The first year in London was strange. It was all so disorganised and my mood was very up and down. I struggled to deal with my feelings and often got frustrated when I felt rubbish, but I didn't know why I was feeling low.

To begin with, I moved in with my new boyfriend Will; we'd been seeing each other for a few months over the summer. His family welcomed me into their home like I was one of them. They were brilliant and let me stay rent-free until I found a flat in London. It was a huge change from living with my dad. I had gone from living pretty much on my own, to living with a family who cared about what I was doing in the evenings and were interested in my day-to-day life.

Will's family had a set mealtime, which definitely helped me stay on top of my eating, although I did put on weight that year. And, very gradually, I began to realise that exercising wasn't everything. Doing less exercise also meant I began to enjoy it much more, something that I didn't even realise was possible.

I don't think Will's family will ever really know how those set mealtimes – and making them such friendly, family times – really helped me stay on top of my eating. So I enjoyed living there, and as they lived right on the edge of Richmond Park, I was able to enjoy endless runs around the park, which I loved.

After a few weeks at Will's parents' house, I moved in with Dan – he was part of our wider friendship group at university and had lived with Will for two years. Dan was tidy, friendly and friends with Will. So we all re-lived our university years while still trying to work for a living! We went out a lot on the weekends and stayed up late in the week.

I was tired a lot of the time, and as we got closer to Christmas, I started to have some issues with my stomach. I ended up having a tummy scan to try and work it out. They put it down to stress, but I assumed that my anorexia may have had a more long-term effect on my internal organs than I thought.

Apart from that blip, life seemed almost normal. There were the usual ups: I started to learn how to fit my running into my schedule better. And the usual downs: I kept pushing people away. But overall, I was doing okay. By the next summer, I realised I wasn't happy with the weight I'd put on and began to squeeze a bit more exercise in. I just wanted to get back to the weight I had been at university.

Mum and I were starting to speak again, and I tried to be more open with her. I don't know why I was struggling with my weight. Maybe I had agreed with Anorexia that I would never go above a BMI of 19. Or maybe it was because I had found aspects of the year tough and decided to concentrate on my weight to help pull me through.

I'd been working in the recruitment industry. The people were great, but I knew this wasn't what I wanted to do with my whole life. And I struggled with not having a plan.

I was keen to do more, and I felt another voice stirring in me. Not Anorexia this time, but the desire to help and support others. I arranged to go to Thailand in October, left my recruitment job and spent the rest of the summer working in a clothes shop. I had always enjoyed shop work, spending time with people, and helping others feel good about themselves.

One day, a girl came in who was quite overweight. She looked so upset. I had a flashback to endless shopping days with my mum and the time I had dragged her out to get a coat I wanted. I bought it and immediately regretted it. I hated the picture in the mirror that stared back at me. The coat made me look fat. Someone at school even commented that it wasn't very flattering, so I never wore the coat again. It hurt that someone could be so mean, but I suppose they'd been right.

I didn't want this young girl to feel what I did, so that afternoon, I went above and beyond to help her find what she wanted. I complimented her, found her more clothes and did whatever I could to make her feel good about herself. It made me happy making someone else feel good. I knew I didn't want her to get sucked into Anorexia's world of calorie counting and exercise that had sucked me in all those years ago.

On 14th October 2012, I had a farewell lunch with my family, went for one final gym session and headed to the airport. I had always wanted to travel and live abroad, and now that Will had found a teaching job in Thailand, it seemed like the perfect time to go. As we drove to the airport, I was scared I was making the biggest mistake of my life. It wasn't as if it was meticulously planned. I hadn't arranged a job out there; I was just winging it. But what if I couldn't find anything? What if the food was hard? How would I know what to eat?

There was no turning back. As we boarded the plane, feeling scared of what to expect, part of me was excited too. I was so good at running away from things, and this time I was running a little bit further ...

CHAPTER 17

RUNNING FURTHER ...

The heat and the humidity hit me as soon as I got off the plane. It was unlike anything I'd ever experienced.

Careering around a mad Bangkok in the back of a taxi, I knew I was way out of my comfort zone. But after a few days of feeling overwhelmed, I decided to pull myself together and contact a nearby children's centre, Mercy International. They were happy for me to volunteer, and in the end I spent a year with them, working with children. The best parts were all the hugs and the sleepovers, although trying to get twenty excited children washed and ready for bed was hard work. We'd often end up flooding the bathroom with water fights, and sometimes I'd have to give out extra treats to bribe them to go to bed. I didn't even care that I had headlice for the entire year. It was all so much fun!

My evenings were spent back in our room, complete with non-flushing toilet. I had to use a fan to keep cool at night and there wasn't any hot water, but I didn't care. It was fun, and it only cost £60 a month! I was still managing to get in some running and sprint training too. I was enjoying myself. I loved the way of life, the people, the food, everything.

At weekends, Will and I would head off to see elephants, explore markets, and take in the wonders of the world. I loved every moment of it.

After a few months, I did occasionally worry about my weight, but the only way I had to weigh myself was by using the scales outside the local 7/11 shop, as early in the morning as possible. I didn't feel the need to weigh myself every week; every fortnight was enough, just so I still felt in control.

It was frustrating that I didn't have a realistic body image. Even today, it is so distorted that when I look in the mirror, I don't always see an accurate picture of myself staring back. Some people can see themselves clearly, or can at least judge their weight by an objective measure, like whether or not their jeans fit. But that's never worked for me.

One of the most life-changing moments for me that year was when John, the head of the orphanage, invited me to come to the Bangkok slums and collect a baby whose mother didn't want him. I really didn't know what to expect. When we went into the children's centre, there were kids fast asleep on mattresses, fans pointing at them as they sweated in the heat. We met the lady who didn't want her child. She was younger than me and was onto her second child. I held him close to me the entire way back to the orphanage and named him Joshua. I loved him and didn't want to let go. John told me I mustn't become too attached, but it was so hard. I found it hard with all the children I worked with. I know I wasn't supposed to, but I couldn't help but let them into my life. I felt so much for them and wanted to do everything I could to make their lives better. I was devastated when my visa ran out and I had to leave.

Before we headed home, Will and I spent a few months experiencing the wonders of South East Asia. I was certainly feeling more relaxed about food. Will enjoyed exercising too, so we went for the occasional run and found a couple of gyms to use. I was doing just enough to keep me healthy, without feeling like I needed to obsess about exercise. More and more, I was starting to see it as an enjoyable part of my life.

I was nervous about coming home and finding a job, but I was genuinely excited to see Mum again. Our relationship had flourished over that year. I had emailed her and Skyped her lots, and I was so pleased our relationship was back on track.

My initial panic over food had settled down – I realised that I would never be able to tell how many calories were in any sort of street food, and it was pleasantly refreshing not being tied down by the calorie counting that had guided me through university. While at times I was still nervous, and didn't know if I'd had too much or not enough, I soon learnt to relax and enjoy my time there. I listened to my body more, and let it guide me as to when to eat. It had been a scary prospect, but I felt like I'd conquered a lot of scary situations and survived.

A few days before I was due to fly back to London, I stumbled across a post on Facebook about a girl called Laura who had passed away as a result of her anorexia. I had lived with Laura in hospital. And now she was dead. I couldn't believe it. Someone so young had actually died from not eating. Did that mean she had succeeded? Had she been a better anorexic than me?

I thought back to all those seemingly empty threats I'd heard in the hospital about the strain I was putting on my body – they could have been true after all. I wonder how many more days I could have gone on without food. And I wondered how Laura's best friend, her anorexia, could actually kill her.

In hospital, we always used to say that, statistically, one of the four of us in a room at any one time would die. And now it had actually happened!

CHAPTER 18

PUSHING MY LIMITS

After a final week in Hong Kong, I headed home to Bristol to begin my job search and try to work out what I really wanted to do with my life. Mum met me at the station, took one look at me and booked me in to see her hairdresser! A Thai lady in the orphanage had dyed my hair to help get rid of the headlice. It didn't work anyway and I'd spent most evenings combing my hair with a nit comb. The dye wasn't really designed for hair like mine and it had turned my hair a sort of tiger colour. I hadn't cared at all while I'd been travelling, but now I wanted a job and I was going to have to look a bit more presentable.

I was lucky to get an internship, which quickly turned into a temporary job at UNICEF, so I was able to continue getting experience of working for a charity and making a difference. However lame that sounds, I knew it was what I wanted to do with my life now. After a year at UNICEF, I headed on for a new challenge at Alzheimer's Society. I was always nervous about new environments when in recovery, worrying whether people would comment on things, whether staff would take lunch in or if they'd go out for lunch all the time. Sometimes it frustrated me that my brain worked like this, but each day made me stronger.

I felt that my eating and my thoughts about food were in a much better place after coming back. But I was still worried about managing my exercise; it felt like that was going to be my greatest challenge. I knew it would be hard not to get sucked back into the Western way of life, and all the obsessions about looking the best, having the best abs etc. I often wondered how much exercise was too much, but was never entirely sure of the answer.

In December 2014, I decided I wanted to test myself by running the Brighton Marathon. I knew that I would have to be careful, but I felt that I was in a good enough place to do it. I wanted to be proactive and make sure I was able to manage it safely, so I downloaded a plan and managed my eating and nutrition carefully. I even had people close to me check in and help me stick to my targets. My rule was that if I lost weight, I would have to pull out. I knew no one was happy about me doing the marathon, so that helped me stay well.

After months of training – and learning to love carbs (they would help fuel me round the course) – I stood at the start line of the Brighton Marathon. Everything I had worked towards over the last six months had led to this moment. I had already achieved the biggest target – staying well – but I knew that I really wanted to do well in the marathon. I set off a bit too quickly, but everything kicked into place and I crossed the finish line in three hours and twenty-six minutes.

The last half had been a bit of a blur, but as I crossed the finish line, I didn't care about anything else. I had done it. I'd nailed the time, and I was so, so happy. A wave of emotion flooded over me, but it wasn't just the achievement. In the run up to the marathon I had tried to be more open about my anorexia and my compulsion to exercise. I was nervous when I was contacted by the *Brighton Argus* newspaper who asked to cover my story, but I'd agreed. I didn't want to feel ashamed about having a mental health problem any more and I wasn't going to worry if people found out.

I have always been driven to do well, and it's the challenges that I set for myself that have helped me stay well. When you're in recovery from a mental illness, it's often the little accomplishments that you value the most. I remember when I ate my first few meals out after leaving hospital ... days when I didn't calorie count, days when I didn't work out ... It was exciting looking back over those achievements, even when a part of me still felt guilty that I hadn't lost loads of weight preparing for the marathon.

I still find it hard not to be ashamed of having a mental health problem. Maybe because it is just so hard to explain. People don't know how to respond when I talk about my issues. And inevitably, the first thing they do is look me up and down to see if I look like I have an eating disorder. My grandma once told me that she was pleased when she looked at me and couldn't tell I had an eating disorder. That was a tough thing to hear, and I don't really know why. Why would I want to look like I was about to drop dead at any moment with my bones stuck out everyone? And I guess that's why, when people say 'you look healthy', it makes me feel a bit funny! It just makes me wonder, does healthy mean fat?

I started to learn the importance of talking about my feelings, so that if I was annoyed or upset, or if I just felt like giving up, I could talk to someone instead of channelling the pain into exercise. Anorexia is normally such a secretive thing, and for some it is a sign of inexpressible sadness. I feel lucky that I got help when I did, and it has just convinced me how important it is that people keep talking.

After the Brighton Marathon, I was nervous that my weight would shoot straight up because I wouldn't be running as much. Luckily it didn't, but if you've ever been friends with Anorexia, you feel like you can never stop the thoughts. I think many people feel the pressure to maintain a certain weight without fixating on it day and night, but when you're an anorexic, everything is a potential trigger.

I know that it is easier to try to numb the pain so you don't feel anything; I'm an expert at it! But I also know that the instant feeling of contentment you get from not eating doesn't last long. Eventually missing one snack or one meal isn't enough. Then you have to do more, and more, and more ... until there's nothing left.

Being controlled by my "best friend", being so close to death, and losing friends to anorexia has made me even more determined to stop anyone else following my path. Now, at last, it feels like things are changing, and people are starting to be a bit more open to the idea of talking about mental health issues.

I wanted to speak out about my issues too, and try to help people see that having anorexia doesn't make you weird. So I began to share my story online, and was invited to speak about anorexia on BBC radio.

There's no two ways about it – it sucks having a mental health problem. And it sucks being scared that one day it might come back. But acknowledging you have a problem is the way forward. As soon as you give your issue a name, it helps lift its hold over you and gives you the power to expose it for what it is.

It may not sound like much of a mantra, but sometimes you just have to embrace those feelings of shit-ness!

Do the things that help make you feel better. When I have a bad day, I always text Mum. The message is simple: "I feel huge," or "I feel awful,' or "I can't go on." My frustration and my anger comes over loud and clear, and sometimes, just saying how I really feel – mask down – helps me feel more in control.

Yes, I still find it hard to talk about it, and I get scared if I feel like I'm letting people down. But as long as I don't let Anorexia beat me, I know that I won't disappoint anyone.

Although it had helped me stay well when I was struggling, I knew that exercise was now my biggest challenge. I used to feel like it couldn't ever let me down, but there had been too many times when I'd head off for a run, feeling utterly alone and trapped within myself. And that didn't make me feel better about anything; it just frustrated me and left me feeling mentally and physically exhausted.

I had to manage my exercise carefully after the marathon. My bones weren't in a good way after years of not eating, and my knees were often sore because of my excessive running, so I had to find other ways of exercising. I found a plan involving weights.

If you struggle with exercise, find a plan that works for you and make sure you give yourself some rest days. I guarantee you will feel altogether better.

Switching off from calorie counting is liberating, although I'm still scared of falling back into my old ways. If only I could just forget how many calories were in everything! But when you've been an anorexic, you can't just switch it off – not when you've spent years researching and learning the calorific content of everything.

After I'd been so liberated with food in Thailand, it was depressingly easy to slip back into the old hospital routine. It was almost as if I had to, because if I didn't, Anorexia would settle back into the driving seat. And just thinking of her could make me second-guess myself. Maybe the calorie counting wasn't so bad after all …

No. Deep down I knew that was a stupid way to think. I needed to test myself more. I needed to push my boundaries. I couldn't let my life go back to being governed by food now. It simply wasn't an option.

I felt nervous excitement as I branched out. Even little things like slicing my own bread instead of having thin-cut slices empowered me. Little victories led to more. It was okay to have an occasional pudding if I was eating out. Terrifying, yes, but worth it.

Rationally, I knew that because I worked out so much, I could afford to eat whatever I wanted. But if that was true, why did I still struggle so much? Anorexia niggled at me after the marathon and questioned my faithfulness to her. She told me I could have run faster if I'd been skinnier, and that I'd get fat if I didn't keep running as much as I could. She said I was a failure; that no one else really cared about me or understood me. I tried reasoning with her; I said my life was better without her. And I reminded her how lucky I was to be alive, no thanks to her.

It isn't always plain sailing, but on your lowest days, you need to remind yourself what Anorexia brings to your life: just pain, suffering and self-loathing.

CHAPTER 19

STARTING TO SLIP

Turning your back on Anorexia is like trying to kick a bad habit. Anorexia doesn't want you to give her up, so she waits for her chance to sneak back into your life when your defences are down. I often felt her trying to befriend me again, telling me what was right and wrong. She always thought she knew best. But I can tell you that the longer I fought her, and the more I pushed her away, the easier it got.

Some battles are harder than others, though. 2016 has been one of the hardest years since my recovery. I felt Anorexia fighting back strongly, guilt-tripping me and making me feel huge again. It wasn't fair. She had been quiet for so long. Why had she suddenly decided to come back and haunt me? Perhaps it was my fault? Was I just too weak to keep going after everything that had happened to me?

I'm not even sure where it all started to go so wrong, but I know things began to escalate pretty fast. One Friday in March I went up to see my maternal grandma at her home. Her dementia was getting pretty bad and I wanted to spend as much time with her as possible.

Grandma had been a very important part of my life. She was such an inspirational lady and I loved her so much. Grandma wrote all the things she had to remember in her diary and rehearsed them, so she wouldn't forget. She would exhaust herself maintaining her part of a conversation, and filled her days with memory exercises which she devised especially for herself. She was a real fighter, a stubborn, determined, caring woman – and I like to think that's how I got my passion and my fighting spirit.

That day, we lay on the bed with the cat and read poetry. It was a good day. She was mostly in a decent mood, and although she didn't know who I was, I was pleased that I'd visited her. It made me laugh when I deliberately left out words and she would stop me. I left that day feeling happy, and I knew those happy feelings would stay with her even if the memories didn't.

Going home, I reminded myself of the other happy times we'd shared, like the summer before when we'd gone to her favourite restaurant and she'd ordered a huge meringue for Will's dessert and he'd been too embarrassed to say he didn't want it. She'd told me she was proud of me and she didn't see me as someone who was consumed by anorexia, but someone who was growing up.

I already missed the woman she had been. I missed the honest conversations and the endless letters we used to send each other. I sat on the train back to London that evening and I cried to myself.

My grandma had tried to fight her Alzheimer's for so long. But a week later, she was put in a care home. I told Mum I wasn't happy about it; no home would be dementia-friendly enough for Grandma. I was actually working for the Alzheimer's Society at the time, and I felt I knew better than anyone else did.

I was nervous when I went to visit her in the home, and as soon as we walked through the door, I knew I hated her being in there. It was a terrible visit. She lay there, a crumpled mess, confused and lost, and had no idea where she was or who I was. I sewed her name onto two new jumpers Mum had brought her, but I had no words. I couldn't even face reading to her. I just wanted her to tell me to leave.

I couldn't bear feeling so helpless. I didn't know why I was struggling to pull myself together. I knew how to act around older people, but I just couldn't do this. I was cross with my grandma for giving up, and cross because I felt like the care home staff weren't spending enough time with her.

The relief flooded over me when we left. And of course, I felt guilty that I was so relieved to get out of there, but I promised myself it would be better next time. I tried to apologise to Mum, but I couldn't even face that. My emotions were getting the better of me again and I tried to revert to boxing-up-my-emotions mode, pretending like I was fine.

By the time I got on the train to London, I was drained. My resolve crumbled and I cried uncontrollably. I didn't know how to cope with my feelings anymore. I told myself not to panic. I repeated the mantra that next time would be better. The initial shock of seeing her in a care home, looking crumpled, small and alone ... that would be gone next time. I would be more prepared. I would be able to face her and have fun. Next time.

There was no next time.

The following Tuesday I got a call from my mum saying Grandma wasn't doing very well. She told me not to worry, but she'd let me know if things got worse overnight. On Wednesday morning, I got up early, went for a run and pushed myself hard. I told myself if I did well on my run, if I ran a certain number of miles in a certain time, my grandma would be okay. I knew I could predict the outcome of things if I ran a certain distance. I'd done it when I wanted a new job after I got back from Thailand, and sure enough, I had run well and got the job I wanted. Surely it would work for my grandma now? Surely if I just pushed myself that little bit harder, everything would be okay?

I struggled to focus at work that morning, and at 10 am the call came through from Mum telling me to come to Didcot. I panicked. I didn't even know how to get from my job in Tower Hill to Paddington, and that was so unlike me. I've always had a weird obsession with transport and the Tube system. I can tell you the best way to get anywhere ... but at that moment, my mind went blank.

I had to text a friend for directions. She didn't even know I'd left work. I hadn't felt able to tell anyone, so I'd just gone without saying a word. I sat on the Tube, tears streaming down my face. A young man opposite me gave me some tissues and asked if I was okay. I dashed through Paddington station, my heart racing, and I got the next train to Didcot. My usual resolve came back. I pushed my feelings away, and through the tears I emailed people at work, apologising that I'd left in a hurry as I'd been feeling unwell.

The train wasn't going fast enough! It was so frustrating. *Come on, Grandma. Hang in there! Please don't go anywhere. I need to see you, to apologise for my last visit.*

Kate met me at the station and we arrived at the hospital to see Mum and Mollie in the waiting room. I just knew. The room felt as if it had had all the life sucked out of it. James and Samuel arrived and the care home manager asked if we wanted to see her.

To this day, I can't get that image out of my head. The woman we saw lying on the bed was not my grandma. It couldn't be her. I felt the guilt coursing through me. The last time I'd seen her had been so awful, and now she was gone. She must have remembered the feelings she'd been left with after my visit.

We just stood there staring, unable to draw ourselves away. If only I had pushed myself harder when I'd been running. If only I had made more effort the last time I'd visited. When I'd been unwell, Grandma had always known exactly what to say to me. I was so angry at myself. And angry that I hadn't been able to have one more meaningful visit with her. I spent time with people affected by dementia all the time, but I hadn't had that time with my grandma.

When she'd gone, I could feel myself slipping back to rock bottom. Nothing made me happy any more. I would find myself weeping quietly on my way to and from work. And then I'd reapply my make-up and push the emotions back into their box. I talked and talked at work – I did whatever I could to keep myself busy, just so I wouldn't have a moment to think about Grandma. But as soon as I was alone and left with my thoughts, the emotions flooded back.

(April 2016)

Dear Grandma,

Aunty Margaret sent me your letters today. I loved them, and I loved how you kept every single one I wrote – even the silly ones. Did you even know what LOL meant when I wrote that down? Looking back and reading them reminded me that you were my absolute rock. Through thick and thin you were there for me, not judging me but supporting me, and I never properly thanked you for that. You listened to my worries while I was in hospital; you were there at the end of the phone when my heart nearly stopped and I felt so afraid that I was about to die. And you were there when I didn't know how to stay well. You held my hand when I needed you most and I am so, so sorry that I found it hard to support you through your dementia (even though I can hear you now telling me off for calling it that)!

I was so proud of you when I came a year and a half ago and you were trying to fight the Alzheimer's. We sat in the conservatory and did Sudoku together, remembering the past.

I am so sorry I couldn't come down and see you more. I wish I had quit my job and moved in with you to look after you, but it just wouldn't have worked. I loved my day with you when I persuaded you to come outside (even though you were so difficult) and we sat in the sun, soaking it up, and I felt like it was us again. I felt like I could talk to you for hours, just like the old days.

I feel like a complete failure even months after you left me. I couldn't cope on that last visit with you – I beat myself up every day about it. I replay it in my mind, and wish I'd known what to say. I wish I had read to you like I did the time before. I wish I had spoken to you and tried to be honest, but I couldn't – and I felt awful that I was so relieved when you told me to leave.

Why did you have to leave me so quickly after that? You should have given me one more chance to be there for you. You were my support and I completely let you down. I am so, so sorry. People always ask what regrets you have in life and that is my biggest regret. Even after everything I've been through, perhaps that is my only regret.

Since you left me, there has been a huge hole in me, a hole which no one else can fill. I struggle to know where to turn and I am so unhappy. I need you back and I need you to shake me. All I want to do is get into your bed and lie next to you, like I used to, with you reading and stroking my hair, taking away all the pain of the world.

I need you to kick me into shape with my eating and I need you to tell me everything about the anti-depressant stuff the GP wants me to take. I Google it all the time and was meant to start it already, but I just can't make myself, especially when I feel like other people aren't happy with me about it.

I hope you can forgive me for being completely awful at supporting you in your last few weeks.

I love you Grandma!

CHAPTER 20

FLIRTING WITH ANOREXIA

Relapse is not a sign of weakness if you fight it.

Hope's mum:

This has not been an easy twelve months for us. My mother, Hope's grandma, died in March 2016, after two and a half years living with Alzheimer's. Her decline became more rapid in February and she was admitted to a care home, where she died just weeks later. Combined with the issues I was having re-applying for my job, and Mollie going through her A Levels, it was a stressful time. Added to that, I couldn't quite believe that I was going to finish childcare after twenty-nine years.

Suddenly in May, I became aware that Hope had lost a lot of weight again. We had an open conversation and she agreed that she would get help. I was worried about her – of course I was – but somehow, it felt different this time ...

Hope:

I was struggling. Grandma had died and I longed for some comfort; someone to be with me permanently. Or just something to make me feel better, but nothing was working. My friends, family and boyfriend Will all rallied round me, trying to do whatever they could. They planned days out to distract me, cinema trips, anything that would help me get through the grieving process. But none of it worked. I was struggling to snap myself out of it. I felt lost, alone and empty. And, as my mood got lower, I could see that I was starting to annoy the people around me. But I was tired of pretending I was okay. I wasn't okay. I was slipping and I knew I couldn't keep going for long.

This was the tipping point. I felt like I'd been through so much and lost so many people over the last few years and now, at last, it was all bubbling to the surface. I began to doubt myself. Had I ever really been okay? Or was I still just a functioning anorexic? I reasoned with myself, saying that people reacted to grief differently, but maybe I just hadn't let myself grieve properly this time? My way of coping was to fling myself into my work. So I went back to work the Monday after she had left me, and made myself feel okay.

I didn't know what would have made me feel better. I just missed Grandma so much and kept flashing back to the last time I saw her. I couldn't shake the feeling that maybe, if I had run harder that day, none of this would have happened.

I thought over my history and remembered how numb I used to feel, how easy it had been to box things up when my emotions got too much for me. But I couldn't do it this time. Why? Every time I tried, I got sucked into that image of her lying there. The guilt was eating me up. Nothing was working. I was frustrated and I couldn't bear feeling like this. I pushed myself harder in the gym and signed up for a half marathon in the hope that it would switch off the feelings.

I was emotionally and physically tired from pushing myself relentlessly through one day after another. My mind began to fall back into all the old thinking traps. I thought back to the days when Anorexia had been there. She had made me feel better. She had helped numb my unhappy feelings and distract me from the pain and the grief. I wanted that comfort again. And I knew she was waiting for me to reach out to her.

She was so seductive. I longed for her to take all the pain away. *She could fix me, I thought. Maybe I could give in to her this time. Just for a bit ...*

And that's all it took to be consumed by her again. My best friend, who I had ignored for so long, was back. She understood me like no one else did. I said I was sorry and told her I remembered everything she had taught me.

I called out to her more and more. I began counting calories again, started exercising more, and weighed myself whenever I got the chance. I was doing it again – shutting myself off and boxing my feelings away, too afraid of would what happen if they exploded all around me. Distracting myself with calories was a wonderful relief from all my emotions.

But underneath the superficial sense of calm, I was scared of her ability to seduce me so easily. And even as I began to skip meals and exercise more, I knew it was wrong. As my body began to shut down again, my periods stopped and I began to shut people out. Just like before.

I can't imagine how hard it is for the people who love you and trust you to watch you submit to Anorexia. I didn't want to hurt them, and I didn't want to risk losing their love and support, so I stopped talking about my feelings and boxed them all up.

I carried on flirting with Anorexia a bit. I let her help me now and then, but I didn't want to get ill. I was terrified that I was just spiralling back into life in a mental health hospital. Why the hell would I want to end up back there ever again? Anorexia had nearly destroyed me last time. She had taken me away from the people who loved me and forced them to watch me slowly killing myself.

I was angry at myself for letting her back in, but I was angrier with her. She had preyed on my vulnerability and loneliness. My best friend was the same manipulative, self-centred, arrogant bitch who thought she knew what was best for me.

I knew I couldn't let it happen. It was time to stand tall, rely on all my stubbornness and fight her head on! So I did something that took every single ounce of courage in me. I called the Mental Health Trust in South West London and cried out for help.

I remember it vividly. I had spent the afternoon talking to one of the operations managers, Karen, about dementia and mental health. She said she knew mental health issues were hard, but everyone had a choice. I was angry at her for saying that, and I didn't think she understood at all ... But then, underneath the anger, I realised she was right. The operations manager saved me that day.

I had a choice to fight my anorexia and I was going to do it. I didn't tell anyone. No one else needed to know or worry. This time, I knew I was strong enough to beat her.

I called the hospital on my way back home. I was so proud of myself for doing it. I had stuff in my life to be happy about. I had so much more to lose this time. And I was determined. I had preached for years about mental health, campaigned for a better balance between the emphasis on physical health and mental health and I had pushed for people to open up about mental health issues. In short, it was time for me to practise what I preached.

I spoke to a lovely administrator who talked me through the process. I booked an appointment with my GP and got a referral to the mental health hospital within six weeks.

I knew it was going to be a long six weeks. I was going through such a low, I didn't know how I was going to stay well; I didn't even know if I had the strength to fight. The weeks that followed were hard work and I sank right back into comfortable, old habits. I started to feel guilty if I didn't work out hard enough. My whole body ached. I felt trapped and didn't know where to turn – if only because I didn't want anyone to worry about me and what I was going through. It was my job to sort this out. I told myself that I didn't care about over-exercising but I had to eat enough. So, I had to track everything – it was the only way I knew I'd stick to it. And I did just that.

One evening my mum took me shopping for my birthday, but there was no part of me that felt any excitement. She sat in the changing room while I got measured, and then she brought up my weight loss and my mood. My mind began to spin and the tears whirled in my eyes. I broke down and told her I'd let Anorexia back into my life.

I can't imagine what it must have been like for Mum to hear that. She couldn't understand how Anorexia could be my best friend; she only saw the pain it brought to our lives. She couldn't feel the reassurance Anorexia gave me; she could only see her daughter slowly wasting away.

I knew she'd be devastated, but I knew that the whole family would be behind me. We all understood so much more about my anorexia now. I had other coping mechanisms too. I took out my eating disorder box and reminded myself of the things people had said about me – that I was a survivor and a fighter. It still helped me to hear that. I looked at my motivation cards; they had brought me so far, and now, because I had stayed well, I had been able to travel, and I had been able to help other people ...

I didn't think I deserved to be sick again, but I knew getting better was going to be up to me. It was my choice. And that was the difference. When I'd been sick before, I didn't feel like I'd had that choice. I had just given in to Anorexia and let her win. But this time around I wasn't going to let that happen. I battled night and day.

A week later, I refused to eat out for my younger brother's birthday and just went home. I was still eating, but I just couldn't face eating out. I was so frustrated at myself and I knew Mum was worried, so she agreed to come with me to my hospital appointment. My BMI wasn't massively under, but that only made things harder – I wasn't going to be thin enough for a quick referral and I wouldn't be eligible for any extra support. Instead, it all relied on me being honest. As I opened up to the hospital staff about my relapse, my calorie counting, my exercise, and the feelings I battled each morning, I felt like I was cheating on Anorexia. She had been there for me after my grandma died; she had been there when I felt all that guilt. She grieved with me and reassured me when no one else could. She knew I needed her, but the doctor was candid. This time, I would probably die if I didn't fight. My body just couldn't go through it all over again.

I relied on Mum to check in on my weight, and my older sister, Kate, would text me throughout the day to make sure I had eaten all my meals. It sounds so simple, but these little interventions were just what I needed. Having a few weeks of someone else supporting me like that gave me the strength I needed to fight. Weirdly, when you have an eating disorder, it feels so much better when someone tells you to eat than if you try to make yourself eat.

Each day brought its own challenges. There were no certainties. And things only got harder ...

CHAPTER 21

READY TO DIE?

On a beautiful day in June, I felt as if my fight was over. I was ready to give up.

Too much had happened and I was too tired to go on. It really was that simple. There was no big revelation or epiphany. I just felt as if I had lost. She had come back into my life and I had been powerless to stop her.

I walked back to Waterloo after work. It was a nice evening and I was still able to enjoy the walk down by the river. The South Bank in the summer was beautiful and vibrant. I used to like watching people and wonder where they were going and what they were doing. They all had stories to tell.

The walk gave me time to think. It would normally have taken about forty-five minutes, but I stopped several times along the way to look into the Thames. I thought back over my last year. I still didn't know what I wanted. I knew my resolve was hanging by a thread now; I felt how very easy it would be to give in to her once and for all. When I got to Waterloo, I sat on the platform. The trains were hot and I was tired. I was tired of everything now. Tired of the mask I wore every day. Tired of the usual routine. Tired of the thoughts.

I sat and watched people dashing to and from their trains, rushing to get home. What did they feel? Had they had a good day?

How many of them were battling with feelings of worthlessness? How many were sad? How many were breaking inside? How did they cope? Where did they find the strength to go on?

I thought back all those years to the night I'd gone with my dad to look for James – back when Anorexia had worked her way into my life and helped me numb the pain.

I thought about what I had achieved in the last three years. If I died now, how would I be remembered? Probably for my running, my work ethic, my caring attitude ... Would people come to my funeral? Would they be sad, or would they actually be better off without me?

I carried on sitting there. I knew then that I wanted to die. It made sense. Life would be better for everyone after I was gone. They wouldn't have to worry any more.

I could picture it. I could see myself jumping in front of the train. I wanted an end to it. I wanted to feel nothing.

I knew I couldn't keep doing this day after day. I'd had suicidal thoughts before, but never to this extent. I thought back to hospital when I had decided I would rather die than be fat. But now, I thought I would rather die than feel anything at all.

I thought about my baby sister, Mollie. She was just doing her A Levels, and I was so excited about the thought of her moving to London. Would Mollie hate me forever if I killed myself?

It's funny the things that go through your mind when you're considering ending your life. But I couldn't go through with it. Perhaps it was my strange obsession with South West Trains; I couldn't stop thinking how annoying it would be for other commuters who would want to get home. I had always told myself I wouldn't be that person.

I texted a friend who was finding life tough too, and I made a deal with her that neither of us would kill ourselves. We made that promise to each other. I didn't know if I believed it, but I do know it stopped me killing myself that day. I reminded myself that there were so many people who cared for me and valued me. It made me feel loved. It buoyed me up.

After that, I got on the train home as if nothing had happened. I boxed it up, went home and cooked dinner. I didn't feel able to tell anyone other than Kate about what had happened. I had never felt that low in my whole life but the main thing was I had fought the desire to kill myself.

When you take a stand and make that decision not to kill yourself, life gets simpler. Doesn't it?

I didn't lie to you. When I made that decision on the train platform not to kill myself, I passionately believed that I was going to stick to it. But that didn't mean it was easy. On that day, I stepped back and walked away. I even made a pact with my friend that neither of us would take our lives. But I was still trapped by those feelings.

After that, every time I stepped on the railway platform, the same dark thoughts flooded my mind.

Life will be better for everyone if I'm not around. No one will have to worry about me anymore. They can get on with their lives and move forward with everything they want to do.

I had made my decision not to jump, but that didn't magically send the thoughts away. And the more I thought about ending my life, the more real it all felt. More than anything, what held me back from doing it was the worry about what it would do to Mollie and how it would affect her studies. Even so, I knew I couldn't get through the next few weeks waiting for Mollie to finish her exams without help.

It was for this reason that I found myself sitting in the doctor's surgery one day. All right, I was an emotional mess – but at least I was trying to be practical and forward thinking!

'Can you give me anything to help me feel better?' I asked the doctor, desperate to just feel okay again. It didn't feel like that would ever be possible. She prescribed me Citalopram, but the prospect was terrifying. *Will it make me put on loads of weight?* I wondered. *Will it change my personality?*

It took all of my courage to agree to the prescription, but at that moment I wasn't quite ready to start taking it. Not yet. Not quite.

I had plans to visit Liverpool Street Market on the Sunday of that week and I knew it would be a good distraction. I needed to try to distance myself from my fears. Knowing I needed to take the Citalopram made me feel weak. I hated having to rely on medication for my brain. Why me? It just felt so unfair.

I felt at such a loss. I didn't know what to do. I wanted this positive mindset back, the old me, the fighter and fun-loving person. But it had been lost.

I took the pill, telling myself that if it didn't work in a month, I would come off it. And whatever happened, I would be off them within six months. Convincing myself of this made the whole thing so much easier to justify taking these pills. But I was still absolutely terrified. Would this change me? Was I actually admitting I needed this? I wanted an instant cure, and while deep down I knew that wouldn't happen, I was slightly disappointed when I didn't feel anything.

Straight after taking it, I headed to the gym, trying to remind myself what I had done was okay. I felt so scared and that I had let my family down and everyone around me. I sat on the Tube to Liverpool Street, wondering when it would kick in, wondering whether I would suddenly put on loads and loads of weight, or whether it would change who I was as a person.

As I walked around the market, I felt quite nauseous. This was first of many side effects I was about to face. I couldn't even manage a proper lunch that day, and admittedly my mind loved that. I climbed in to bed that evening before 10 pm, falling straight to sleep. I was relieved I was so tired, but what I didn't expect was to be up at 1 am, wide awake, unable to sleep, pacing around my one-bed flat. I didn't know what to do.

At 2 am my mind was still racing. *The alarm will be going off in four hours.* At 3 am, I thought, *I only have three hours now. Perhaps stretching will help ... Then came 4 am. Why can't I just sleep?*

At some point I must have fallen asleep on the sofa, as the alarm woke me up at 6 am. I was exhausted, but usually I would be at the gym by 6.30 am, so I could fit in my workout before work. After rushing through a quick bowl of porridge, I headed to the gym, still feeling slightly sick.

Why aren't I feeling better? I thought irrationally.

I made it to lunchtime in the office, but I couldn't stay any longer. I felt so unhappy. It was taking every bit of energy I had to try to engage with the world. I texted my manager to say I felt unwell and would try to work from home that afternoon, and then I headed out.

I sat on the edge of the Thames for an hour or so, crying.

The change came slowly. For two weeks I felt miserable, and it was beyond my power to stop it. And then, very gradually, I began to feel a bit better. My reliance on exercise was still out of control, but my mood was beginning to improve. I knew that I had the strength to get back on track; I just had to work out how to do it. After all, I already had the tools I needed.

I began by going back to my meal plans from hospital. At that moment, it felt like the only way to get back on track was to start calorie counting again, even if that meant having a snack every evening before bed. It was frustrating to have to go back to the basics, but I tried to embrace a positive mindset.

And if I could cling onto anything, it was this one thought: I wouldn't let anorexia beat me. I couldn't end up as an outpatient again. That gave me strength, and bit by bit my resilience came back.

I just had to take each day as it came, never planning much beyond that week. At times I still felt empty. I missed my grandma, and I had to fight even harder to get rid of *that* voice in my head. I knew that the more I stuck with it, the better it would be. But it had taken the best part of six months to get there.

I finished writing the first edition of this book in good spirits: I knew I hadn't beaten anorexia, but I felt that I was taking back control over my life. I just didn't know how hard it was going to be to *keep* control.

Those six months were tough. But getting through it made me tougher. Just as well with Christmas around the corner.

Over that summer, I had tried to open up more about my mental health. It hadn't even occurred to me that anyone would have noticed my weight loss, or thought that my usual bubbly self was disappearing. Nikki, one of my best friends, suggested going out for brunch one Friday morning and after the initial pleasantries, plunged right into it. I was shocked that she had noticed, but really touched that she had cared.

She asked me how I had felt. She wanted to know what was going wrong, and asked if I was counting my calories again. For some reason, I couldn't lie to Nikki. I trusted her with the truth. I knew she wouldn't interfere, but would be there for me if I needed her. After that, Nikki decided we would have a summer of fun to help get me through that "hiccup", and she delivered. We had an amazing summer, lots of nights out, lovely meals, cinema trips, the lot.

I know I was very lucky at how accepting of my mental health issues my friends at university had been. And as Nikki had been so brilliant, I decided to tell the rest of our group of girls. I did my matter-of-fact way of talking about it and they accepted it. They were open to the idea and they were there to help me if I needed it.

I felt guilty a lot of the time, especially around those closest to me. I felt like I had let them down. I had failed them. Knowing someone with a mental health problem is tough, and I know that at times I can be a complete nightmare. But opening up to friends and family always helped me back on track.

Work was a different story. At first. For some reason, I have always struggled to be open about my mental health at work. I "mask up" each day, regardless of how I feel, and head into the office. I suppose I was worried that people would judge me, or that it would hold me back in my career.

But I was talking more openly about mental health issues and people were starting to ask why. I started out giving wishy-washy answers until one day when my friend Fionnuala asked me. I gave her the usual anonymous response, but then texted her a blog I had written. I was scared of what she would think, afraid that she wouldn't want to be my friend any more. But she understood, and she has been amazing.

So I decided to open up to some more of my friends at work and Simon, Gavin, Laurie and Tatjana have all stood by me. Now, I don't have to pretend anything. I don't need to "mask up" or say I feel fine if I don't. These are the kinds of friendships I can't live without. And since they have all been so accepting, I have tried to be honest with more people. It hasn't been easy, but sticking to the facts and not going into details about my feelings have helped. And the more people I talk to, the more I discover that everyone seems to have their own story to tell.

Over the last twelve months, I have grown closer to my brothers too. James has been there whenever I have needed him, reminding me to keep battling. Since coming back from Thailand, I have continued to get closer to Mum too. She has been my absolute rock this year. She knows when she needs to sympathise, when she needs to hug me, and when she needs to just let me cry. And sometimes she'll tell me to "gird my loins" and get through the day any way I can.

Over the summer, I called her one day from the corridor at work. I felt completely overwhelmed and didn't know what to do. She let me cry down the phone for about ten minutes before telling me we needed a plan of distraction. We came up with one together, and it gave me the strength to pull myself together and head back into the office. It was hard work wearing that mask throughout the summer, but I managed it. It isn't something I'm proud of, but I think that hiding so much from the people around me helped me to keep going at work and in my day-to-day life.

I am better at making the time to be with my family now, and when we see each other, it is always so much fun. I'm sad that I still struggle with my dad. His busy life is so full, but I can't fault him for it. He stood by me when I was in hospital. I know that even though he has so little time, he still cares about me. In the past, I would have gone straight to Anorexia if Dad didn't get in touch when I wanted him to, but now I feel so far removed from her that I just don't need her. I know her solution isn't a long-term fix and it definitely won't last. I now have my own network of support, good friends and family to help me.

Throughout my year of relapse there were heaps of things that helped make life bearable, from making the most of my job, to organising social things with friends, to trying to be more open with those around me. I started to talk about my feelings and learnt to embrace them. But I also allowed myself to have days when I struggled with my emotions, without punishing myself for it. While I continued to self-destruct, to sabotage some relationships that were getting too close for me, I got better at letting people in too. I got better at sending a quick text in the morning if I felt awful, or just to let someone know I wasn't doing so well. Having a bad day is nothing to be ashamed of, and while you want to be able to get on with your life without getting unwell again, it is important to realise that relapsing isn't a sign of weakness. Failing to fight is the only weakness. If you carry on fighting you can beat it. I know it.

A friend from work said something to me that resonated more strongly than anything else. One evening after I asked him how he managed when things were difficult, he texted me this message:

"I WILL NOT LET THIS BEAT ME."

It was a powerful message, and I felt like it hit the nail on the head. He wasn't trying to tell me everything would be okay. He wasn't making any false promises that I would feel amazing the next day. No, he was being realistic. And I loved that about him. He understood where I was coming from, he knew what it felt like to mask up, and he understood why I was fed up and frustrated when my anorexia bit back at me.

When I wake up, there are days when I use this message to give me strength. Even to this day he has no idea how much his support meant to me at that point in my life, but I am 100% certain that it will stay with me for the rest of my life.

Now I understand that just being a fighter isn't enough. I have to outsmart Anorexia. I need to understand the signs that she is creeping back, so that I can still keep myself well when things get tough.

After Grandma died, I felt uncertainty about my anorexia. Stupidly, I'd signed up to the Richmond Half Marathon. I just thought that if I did it in a super-fast time, it would bring her back. And in that moment, I wanted her back. Even though I was fed up of training, even though I knew I was annoying everyone around me with my obsessions, I somehow thought it would help me feel better. I had my usual pre-race nerves, and I felt terrible most of the way around, but I got a personal best of one hour and thirty-one minutes.

I had lots of friends there, real people who had come out to cheer me on. As I crossed the finish line, I bumped into an old friend: Anorexia. But I knew I didn't need her friendship anymore.

Maybe it's a good thing that I had a mini-relapse, because now I know I can deal with it if it ever happens again. I know that every day I shut Anorexia out is a day that I win. It is a day when I get stronger. And as my friends and family will tell you, I am a driven, determined and ever-so-stubborn person – something that definitely helps me refuse to give in to Anorexia.

I won't let her win again, not ever! I'm a sucker for a cheesy pop song, and cheesy as it may sound, I know that what doesn't kill you makes you stronger.

2016

Dear Anorexia,

You are a manipulative bitch. You tried to come back this year. You got me when I was weak and vulnerable. But I am not going to let you win.

You did nothing for me. Yes, I am amazing at calorie counting and being sneaky with food, but seriously, are they good qualities? It might help in the odd pub quiz, but come on, Anorexia!

You falsely promised me. You falsely held me in the night when I missed my grandma, but she wouldn't want you to be friends with me. And I certainly don't want to be friends with you. You have made me slip into bad habits but I will not let you beat me. I didn't let you beat me last time and I certainly won't let you win now.

Yours, still fighting, still heading onwards and upwards,

Hope

Dear Mum, Dad, Mollie, Kate, James, Samuel and Will,

I will be forever grateful for you standing by me this year. It wasn't easy for you, and I know that. I do sometimes wonder what you think when you look at me. I want to know what is going through your head when you watch me eat, watch television, or even when I let my competitive streak come out and I cheat at board games!

I am sorry for this year. Sorry that, having managed to stay well for so long, I pushed you all away and shut you out when all you wanted to do was help. I am sorry that I am so bad at talking about things and sharing things with you. I am just afraid of you all walking out on me and giving up on me. But you haven't, and I am gradually learning to believe that you never will. I feel so lucky to have you all.

That beautiful day in June, when I felt like giving up, was stupid. I can't explain why I felt like that, but I thought your lives would all be easier if I didn't exist. You wouldn't have to worry about me missing meals, or worry about the future with me – you would never again have to worry about me thinking of killing myself. I remember that day as vividly as if it was yesterday. I played over so many scenarios in my head. I wondered who would be first to know, who would identify me, who would cry the most, and what you would all do without me?

Will, I wondered who would make your breakfast in the mornings and stop you watching labrador videos so that you would go to the gym. Mollie, who would give you all that essential advice about boys? And Kate – you wouldn't have anyone quite as blunt to go shopping with!

I know this year hasn't been easy for any of you. It has been one shit thing after another. Life throws so many challenges at all of us on a daily basis, but I know one thing for sure – we are all as stubborn and determined as each other. None of us will ever give in.

Thank you for putting up with me and coming to appointments with me, Mum. You were an absolute rock – you were always there for me at the end of the phone, even when I was up late at night. When I look back over the last year, you have all been fab, and you have all helped me in your own ways. I can never thank you or my friends enough. You supported me. You didn't promise me the world, but you were always there when I needed you most. Thank you for putting up with my mood swings, my panics, my anxiety and all my silly default settings. Thank you for not giving up on me when all I wanted to do was give up and shut you all out.

I hope that I made you proud. I know I am certainly proud of myself. Proud that I beat fucking Anorexia. She isn't worth it, but you all are!

Love you always,

Hope

CHAPTER 22

AM I JUST A FUNCTIONING ANOREXIC?

'So stand tall against the world and bawl,
A little girl who gets up every time she falls,
See the bigger picture, when I'm gone, I'm gone,
So this is my song,
Head up, and remember – be strong.'

Hope Virgo

Looking back, I still try to find answers as to why I had an eating disorder.

Was it the sexual abuse when I was younger?

Was it because I was crying out for help?

Was it a control thing?

Or was it that I had this biological factor inside me, a gene that made me anorexic?

And I still wonder why I didn't die all those years ago when my heart was so close to stopping.

I spent hours researching and questioning how much of my mental health is dependent on my biology. I felt there must be something in me that made me prone to Anorexia. Or was it just the addictive sense that, having found such an amazing way of switching off from everything, I couldn't stop? Anorexia had sorted me out and made me feel alive, while feeling zero emotion. She had been my best friend for so many years. She'd held me close, loved me, motivated me, and made me feel good (at times!) about myself.

When I have a bad day, I often lie awake at night and think about all the things that have happened to me. I break them down into stages and think about the impact they've had on my life. I beat myself up, wishing I had been assertive and stopped that guy forcing himself onto me. I wish I hadn't let him guilt trip me or take control. But I did. And because of him, and because I felt I couldn't rely on anyone else, I came to believe that I could only ever rely on Anorexia. She would never let me down.

When I was in hospital, I never thought I would get to the point where I would be able to go out for dinner and actually enjoy it. I certainly never thought I would be able to wear a bikini, or have days when I wouldn't work out and still feel happy. Looking back, things have got easier. I remember the times when even a single day of not working out would have flung me into a state of panic, when I used to think that not running for one day would mean putting on weight straightaway. But now that my mind is so much clearer, I can reason with myself, and I know this is silly.

Going from not eating anything and being institutionalised to trying to live a normal life is tough. You lose who you are and you lose any understanding of what "normal" is. There was no switch to make me better, no way to switch my food settings back to normal. It all took time. I'm still working on it. And I think that's okay. My bad days are so few and far between that I can love my life.

I recently went to Jordan for a week and Anorexia was so quiet, she was basically non-existent. It was my first holiday since my relapse and I was scared that I'd be eating out all the time, without any regular exercise. I don't like the fact that I still instinctively think like that. Even though I have achieved so many little victories, it saddens me to think I've lost so much confidence in my ability to stay well ...

But I did it. And I had an amazing week, trekking through the desert, eating whenever there was time, and driving down the desert highways. I laughed a lot and experienced a whole new way of living. I loved every second of it. And I knew then that my life was good. I was lucky, and I didn't want to sacrifice everything I had worked for, just for the chance of being a better best friend to Anorexia.

The first morning at breakfast, all they served was flatbread, omelettes and cheeses. I got a black coffee and sat there overlooking the city. There was the distant echo of the call to prayer and the sound of children chattering down below. I looked down at my plate of flatbread.

Come on, Hope! One meal isn't going to affect your weight.

Try to relax. You want children one day and that won't be possible if you don't stay well.

Live a little!

I opened up to the motivation and pushed Anorexia deep, deep down into the pit of my stomach. Further away from me, much further. I knew I could never ever let her beat me now.

I have lots of days like this now. I can go out and enjoy life, and I can eat what I want without feeling the need to work out. I know that, if I want to go out for dinner and eat and drink what I want, I can. I never thought I would have a day when I didn't feel Anorexia lurking, a day when I didn't feel fat, but now, days like these come around often. I feel no guilt and I switch off completely from her.

I do still have to be careful when I push myself too hard at the gym or miss a meal. Maybe it's inevitable that, as someone who has recovered from an eating disorder, I overthink everything. If I'm ever unwell, I struggle with wondering whether I should or shouldn't eat until a bug passes. I guess that's just the way I am now, but it does sometimes frustrate me that I'm incapable of switching off from my anorexia altogether.

Can you ever really get over a mental illness? Or will it always be there in the back of your mind?

If you have ever known Anorexia, you know what she's like. The people around you think it's easy: just stop exercising quite so much, and eat a bit more. Simple!

But Anorexia cuts so deep. My desire to exercise has bordered on the obsessive. There have been times when I have been jittery and uncomfortable just because I know I'm not going to be able to exercise. There have been days when I have woken up feeling fat, when it doesn't matter what I wear. I will try on one outfit after another and she'll taunt me. 'You can't wear that! Look at the size of your stomach!'

I worry that I still want to compare myself to others. I worry that, when I sit down to eat, I have to stop myself from instinctively adding up all the calories on my plate. I know that I can't ever completely let my guard down because underneath it all, she's still there. But it's like a physical injury; you can learn to live with it.

I still have tendencies to box my emotion up and push people away when the emotions get too much for me to deal with. (Everyone has their coping mechanisms, right?) But I can also subject my thoughts to closer scrutiny. What does it really achieve? Yes, it means that people can't hurt me, and I can't disappoint people, but other than that, it does nothing for me. All it ever did for me in the past was put me in hospital. Objectively, I know that life is so much better when you let people into your life; when you talk about things.

I used to be so secretive about having a mental health problem, and if people found out then I'd push them away or pretend I was 100% cured. But why should I be ashamed? Why am I still ashamed of something that I fought so hard to beat, something that took me so close to death?

Sometimes I worry that being open and honest with people will affect my career. But that has never happened. I sometimes worry that it will make people watch what I eat. But it really doesn't.

People may have strange ideas about mental health just because they don't understand it. Perhaps like I did when I was younger, they imagine scenes of people being strapped down and sedated. But it's not like that at all. And we need to stand up and talk about mental health so we can get rid of that stigma.

There is no definitive research stating that mental health issues are the result of nature or nurture. But I am convinced that eating disorders and mental health aren't rooted in a person's biology. The one thing I do know is that my anorexia has made me who I am today. It has made me determined, and maybe even slightly stubborn. But it has also made me driven and ambitious. It has changed me for the better, and while I still ask why it chose me, I don't think it really matters. It isn't anybody's fault. What's important now is that I take my opportunity to fight it and turn a bad situation into something good.

So at those times when I wake in the morning, take one look in the mirror and hate the girl with that huge tummy staring back at me, I try to remember that these are just thoughts. They are definitely not my reality. And if my mind wanders to exercise, calories and skipping a meal, I know that I am stronger, more stubborn and better equipped to resist.

That doesn't mean it's plain sailing. I don't suppose it will ever be easy. I have read stories of people being miraculously cured of their anorexia, but I know that I am not cured. I still have to work hard at staying well, and I have to be realistic. That is the only way to keep her at bay. On bad days, I still go back to my eating disorder recovery box and remind myself what a fighter I was. What a fighter I still am.

I wish I could tell you that my life has been consistently amazing since being discharged. That is simply not the reality of living with Anorexia. But I can tell you that it has always been worth staying well. I don't ever want to give up fighting Anorexia, and neither should you.

I know how she makes you feel: you think she is your friend; you think she can solve everything and make you feel amazing ... but the reality is, she cannot. Instead she will destroy you and everything around you, piece by piece. I never used to believe people who said that to me. I assumed they were lying; they didn't really get it. But trust me when I tell you, I have lived through the agony of being Anorexia's "best friend" and come out the other side a stronger and happier person.

I have learnt how to manage my life day to day – and I have never lost sight of the reasons why I had to go on fighting. I have come this far and seen the other side. I have had tantalising glimpses of a normal life not governed by food. And the 100% truth is this: life is so much better.

I may be Hope Virgo, functioning anorexic. But more importantly, I am Hope Virgo – survivor.

Dear Mum and Dad,

I don't think I have ever thanked you for the support you gave me throughout my eating disorder.

Firstly, I want to say sorry. Sorry for causing you so much grief, for being such a nightmare to live with and for nearly killing myself. I was weak and you were my strength. Even when I fought back, I am thankful that you didn't give up on me.

Thank you for driving me to CAMHs each week while I sat in a mood in the waiting room.

Thank you for crying with me and celebrating small victories.

But here is what I want to tell you – no matter how hard you try, you will never fully understand what it is like to be living in the midst of an eating disorder. The fear that passes through my mind when I sit down to a meal, the panic that rises in me when I have to socialise around food? That you will never understand.

I would lie there in bed each evening, frantically adding up all my calories throughout the day. I would lie there wondering when I could exercise again, or I would find plastic bags to make myself sick in. I would lie there while the voice of Anorexia grew and grew inside me, beating me up, questioning me on what I had eaten during the day. 'Have you exercised enough? You didn't need that extra snack! They are all trying to make you fat!' She was relentless. She never stopped. And some nights I just couldn't shut her up. Some nights I battled into the night, exercising in my room, letting her rip me to shreds, letting her push me ever closer to death.

I wish that she would leave me alone and stop bullying me. I wish I wouldn't wake up again until she has gone. I know how hard you tried to understand. I appreciate the endless hours of reading, family therapy, all the books and internet searches on anorexia. I am grateful you tried.

At times, I wanted to die. I wanted to give up this fight and let her win. I saw you fall apart. I saw your eyes watching my every move and I saw you battling with yourself. I heard you outside the bathroom listening to me making myself sick; I heard you lingering in the corridor outside my bedroom, deciding whether to come in. I watched you looking on in agony, hurting as my heart slowed down, as Anorexia took over every part of my life.

I am pleased you haven't had to go through this with Anorexia pulling at you and beating you up. I mean that. I couldn't face watching her be this nasty, this manipulative, to someone else.

Am I an eating disorder survivor? Will I ever be completely cured?

I love how you remind me who I am. You don't just see my eating disorder. And you no longer see someone trapped in a deathly cycle; you see me as me. You see a fighter. You believed in me and you still do.

You don't have to understand my past to share in my journey, but simply by holding my hand and being there for me, you can help me get to the finish line.

All my love, Hope

CHAPTER 23

LIVING LIFE ON MY TERMS

Hope's mum:
When Hope started showing signs of anorexia again, she gave me categorical assurances that she did not want to be ill again – and I believed her 100%. She was so much more open about how she was feeling. I realise how very difficult it has been for her, and I am proud of her. She is an incredibly gutsy girl.

Hope:
If one in four people have a mental illness in the UK, that must include some of my friends and some of the people I work with. It must include people you know too.

Maybe they're all afraid to open up, afraid of the stigma. Anorexia is such a secret disease and maybe that's the way she likes it. Maybe she wants to stop us opening up to others. And that's why we have to do just that. That's why we have to talk about her and expose her for what she is.

When I walk down the street, meet someone new, or travel on the Tube, I can spot someone who has had an eating disorder a mile off. I no longer look at them with envy, just with sadness. I had to nearly die before I realised that maybe something was wrong. But now I know the signs of relapse, the signs of slipping. And I know that life is worth fighting for. I don't want to let food govern my existence. Living life with Anorexia, no matter how close you feel to her, or how much you value her, just isn't worth it.

I have lost three friends to mental health problems and I don't want to see more people lose their fight. I promise you that being well and staying well is worth it. It's the sort of life that your secret best friend doesn't want you to have, but it's the life you deserve.

It has been quite a therapeutic experience, writing this book and sharing my story. At times, I felt scared about opening up. I was afraid of the judgement of others and whether it would have a negative impact on me.

But writing every page has reinforced just how determined I am to stay well. And it has made me even more desperate to help others see that they can fight (and beat) their anorexia. I know that having a mental health problem is not a sign of weakness. You just have to make sure you keep fighting it.

Living with Anorexia is definitely not all it is cracked up to be. She promises to be your best friend, but in reality, she is only there to knock you down and manipulate you. Ask yourself, why would a friend who loves you do that?

I am not going to stand here and tell you it is easy! It isn't, especially when you have lived with Anorexia and food governing your life for so long. But God, fighting that nasty manipulative voice in your head is worth it! I can't reiterate that enough!

Even after surviving my mini-relapse, I knew that Anorexia could still resurface again. While this is scary, I know I have ways to manage it. People who know about my eating sometimes ask me how I stay well, and I have developed my own coping mechanisms. The top five things that keep me well are:

- Talking to people
- Keeping active
- Working towards my life goals
- Avoiding triggers
- That box under my bed

I admit that talking to people is something I have struggled with – and still struggle with at times – but identifying people in your life who can support you, people you can text to tell them you're having a bad day, is so important. These are the people who will help you to stay well. If you can have complete trust in these people, they will be your lifeline. They are not there to make you fat, they are there to hold your hand through the good times and the bad. They won't tell you everything is okay when it's not, but they will keep you fighting, day by difficult day.

Just a few months ago, I asked Mum outright if she thought my weight looked okay. We stopped in the middle of central London, and I lifted up my jumper so she could give me an honest answer. I have learnt over the years to trust my mum – and that has taken time – but I'm very lucky to have that level of reassurance. I won't ever forget the times when she'd make me a salad, and I used to check to see if she'd hidden any extra food in there. But now, I completely trust her. So please, let your friends and family rally round you. Cherish their trust. Let them help you, step by step.

Keeping active is important to me, whether that's exercising, making sure I have a quick walk on my lunch break, or socialising with friends. I know I need all of these things in my life. But again, it's a delicate balance between that and managing my own downtime. At my lowest points, I didn't know if I wanted to be around people or not. But trust me when I say that spending time with people always helps. When you are best friends with Anorexia, she isolates you. You might not think she will; you might even think that she is all you need. But it isn't true! She is lying to you. Book some activities you'll enjoy and make sure you take time out to enjoy the company of others. Better yet, combine the two: I have started working out in the park with a work friend before we head into work. And it has helped me rediscover my love of exercise in a non-obsessional way.

I've mentioned the box I keep under my bed. No one ever sees it apart from me and I don't look in it very often. But just knowing it's there for support really helps. All those memories from hospital, my meal motivations, an inspirational book that Kate made me, poems, cards and Tinkerbell dust – it all helps to support me. If I struggle, I remind myself how hard I worked to get well and I read back through all the things I learnt in hospital.

As long as I am working towards my life goals – career, children, travelling and being able to eat out without restrictions – I know that I am in charge of my life, not my anorexia. All of these things matter so much more than my anorexia. They make my life worth living.

Identify your goals and make sure you stick to them. Write them down if you have to, put them in your wallet and don't ever forget them.

Over the last few years I have learnt my triggers – days when I start to count calories, days when I am tempted to exercise too much, or days when I cut out a snack. These things range in extremes, but I know that if I am in control, I will always make the right call. And if I feel like it's all too much and I'm losing control, I'll tell Hope Virgo to pull herself together and stay strong.

I urge you to get to know your triggers, and the people who make your anorexia want to come back. I know that there are people in my life who comment on food far too much, and I need to prepare myself for seeing them. But that way, I know that I can still support them without it impacting me. I know that afterwards, I may need to reassure myself about what I need to do to stay well. So, try to identify these people in your life and decide when you can, or can't, see them. Taking control like this makes you a stronger person.

I love my good days, days when I can get up in the morning, go for a run and really enjoy it. Days when I can go to work, feel happy, and listen to my body decide when I want to eat. These are the days that make life worth living. These are the days that remind me that Anorexia isn't my friend.

Some days are scary. Just a few weeks ago, we went to a food market for lunch. I had chosen what I would have the week before so I wouldn't have to worry about it, but when we arrived, the stall I was expecting wasn't there. I panicked. But I managed. After my initial worrying, I managed to choose something else.

If you're recovering from anorexia – or just thinking about the possibility of recovery – I encourage you to take these small baby steps. Push the boundaries throughout your recovery. It can even be quite exciting. I've found that there is so much food that I used to exclude from my diet altogether that I now love.

Just recently I've actually made a list of foods that I didn't think I would ever touch, and now I'm planning to branch out, to begin eating things like chocolate brownies or fish and chips on the beach. It's still nerve-wracking, but I know I am ready to do it. And above all, I want to do it.

It feels wrong, the first time you start having things if you don't know what their calorific content is, but each time you do it, I guarantee it will get easier. And I can promise you, that wonderful sense of achievement trumps any feelings of guilt.

It feels good to let your guard down. Just a few days ago, I went out with some friends for lunch, had a few drinks in the afternoon, and then enjoyed a cocktail party in the evening. I didn't worry about the food or the weight; I just had a great time with people who genuinely care about me (unlike Anorexia).

It isn't easy to let your guard down all the time, but when you do, it feels amazing. Don't be afraid to start small ...

Try a day without calorie counting, or a day where you eat a tiny bit more, or a day where you just let your guard down, and it will get easier. Baby steps are the way forward! And whatever you do, make sure you talk about things. I know it's hard. I am officially the best person at self-destructing and boxing things up, but that isn't helpful or healthy. Anorexia, my "best friend", nearly killed me. She left me weak, feeble and alone. But now my life is so much better. And my future is mine to decide, not hers.

If you are suffering with anorexia, I hope my story shows you that you can beat it. You can live the life you want. And your life can be amazing.

So stand tall, little girl, and then face the world!

PART 2

STANDING TALLER

CHAPTER 1

SHOULD I HAVE SHARED MY STORY?

So that's me – this was the most honest I have ever been about my journey. But where am I now? Am I fully recovered?

I am a healthy weight now and I eat, so surely that means I am fixed, right? Well, not exactly. Anorexia involves more than being a particular weight or shape. Just because someone looks physically okay, it doesn't mean that everything is okay inside. There are days when I still really struggle with anorexic thinking, when I worry about calories, food, and my weight. This tends to happen when I'm feeling things I don't want to feel, especially pain. I don't know why; I guess no one likes feeling pain. But when I do, I have to be proactive so as not to let the anorexia suck me back in.

Everyone has this image of anorexic people in their heads. It's a picture of someone stick thin and struggling, someone who seemingly has nothing. But anorexia is so much more than that – it is about switching off from day-to-day life, keeping yourself safe when emotions get tough. It isn't about weight or being stick thin. It's about trying to take control of your emotions and manage your feelings. It is about trying to stop hurting when life feels really tough.

Anorexia is part of who I am, yes – and a huge part of who I am – but it doesn't define me. It doesn't make up all of me. This is the only the start of my story. And instead of ruining me, it has made me a fighter, a warrior. And now I have a drive to make a difference.

A few months after my book was first published, someone close to me made a comment about my book. They sent me quite an abrupt message, telling me that they didn't like the fact I was sharing my story and they thought it was slightly too much information. It really hit a nerve. When I decided to share my life in the public domain – a story that for so long had caused me grief, a story of which I had felt completely ashamed – I knew I was going to have to learn to grapple with comments like these. But it still really hurt me. It made me question it all. Had I been selfish? Perhaps I should have thought more about the knock-on effect of having a book about my recovery? Perhaps those around me would be less embarrassed if I hadn't opened up? If I had written a book about breaking my leg, would it have been better for those around me?

But I know now that I shouldn't be embarrassed about it. The truth is, I shouldn't feel ashamed of having had an eating disorder. I shouldn't be ashamed of my relapse. And I shouldn't be ashamed of telling my story.

And besides, I'd always longed to do it. I've always been a very caring person, and I find joy in helping people. So when I started beating Anorexia, I took it on as my life plan to go and fight that battle for others. Publicly. And so, in the following chapters, I'll show you how I've done it.

We must keep fighting stigma. We must get everyone talking about mental health and completely normalise the conversation. If we don't do that, even more people will suffer in silence.

And that is just not acceptable.

CHAPTER 2

IMPOSTER SYNDROME

When the first edition of this book came out in 2016, I was invited to do a lot of media appearances and talks, the first of which was a slot on the Chrissy B Show. We were to film in a warehouse in North London, and honestly, I didn't know what to expect. I was excited about the prospect, but I was so nervous about looking stupid and saying the wrong thing. How long would it take? Would there be a green room? Would I answer the questions properly?

On the way to the studio, I looked down at myself. I had spent ages choosing what to wear, but I still felt slightly uncomfortable, and this sent my brain into overdrive. *Does this dress make me look fat?* I panicked. *What if I can't do this?* I had no idea what Chrissy was going to ask me or how I would respond on camera. But perhaps unsurprisingly, it went fine – although I forgot to include my book title. Tatjana, my resident PR manager, was not happy about that! I knew I had a lot to learn about PR, but thankfully I felt excited about the prospect of what was coming.

As the gigs continued to come in – the next ones occurring at Lincoln University and Henrietta Barnett School in London – I began to realise that I'd found my passion. I realised how much I loved public speaking and offering people hope around recovery. I knew first-hand what it was like to struggle and feel completely isolated and I didn't want anyone to have to go through anything like what I went through.

This was it, my lifetime passion: standing in front of groups of people, helping them, giving them insight into my recovery. Going back to my day job seemed mundane in comparison to actually making a long-term difference in people's lives. I longed for more of this. I was happy that my book was already helping others, but I wanted to do more and more public speaking.

The flurry of media interest continued and I continued to make appearances wherever I could. I gave an interview at BBC Radio Bristol, where I'd first appeared in 2013, and shocked the presenter with my new, grown-up demeanour. I had a photoshoot with the *Daily Mail*, who caked me in make-up to the point where I no longer looked like myself. I was even featured in *Runner's World*, one of my favourite running magazines. They sent me lots of kit to choose from, and we had a fun few hours taking snaps, posing, and running the same 20-metre stretch over and over. It was all so much fun and I loved it. I was doing something I could only have dreamt of doing.

Surely, then, I had made it? Surely, I should have been happy?

But here's the reality.

There still comes the moment when then the magazine arrives in the post and you see the image they've used for the feature ... and you cannot help but scrutinise it. *Do I look big? I fretted. Do I look unfit? Will others look to me for recovery inspiration? Will they see me as a beacon of hope or as someone who has just "let everything go"?*

One of my biggest fears when giving a talk or being interviewed about my book was that people would think I didn't "look" like a person with anorexia. I thrived on appearing in the media, from Sky to *BBC Newsnight* to *Good Morning Britain*, but getting trolled by people stating that I was a "fat anorexic" and "doing things for attention" really fed my insecurities.

I've had those worries in other arenas as well. At one point, I realised how much I wanted to work in hospitals, though I didn't really know for sure whether patients would be open to listening and to changing their thoughts specifically about anorexia. I knew that when I had been unwell, I didn't believe that anyone fully understood what I was going through, and so at the beginning I'd turned hospital staff away. But now I was desperate to be able to show patients that despite it being hard work, you can recover. Of course, I needed to paint an honest picture of it.

And yet, I still somehow felt judged. I was so worried that the people were looking at me thinking I looked fat, thinking that they didn't want to be my size, thinking that I had let myself go. It took all of my energy those first few times to stand my ground. It was like going into battle against Anorexia, but not just mine. I was fighting so many other people's anorexia too.

Learning to manage "imposter syndrome" is very frustrating. I can spend hours thinking I am not good enough at what I do, worrying that others are better, that I look like a "fake anorexic". That's still Anorexia's voice kicking in. *You're a failure, a waste of space. You don't help people at all.* Sometimes it makes me start wondering how many calories I've had that day. And the worst part is that, although my "bad days" are getting fewer and further between, they make me feel hypocritical. They make me wonder whether I should really be doing what I am doing.

Yet despite all this – and despite the fact that being a public speaker about mental health has been challenging at times – the reality is that I have met some amazing people along the way who make it all incredibly rewarding. Some of them are now a real part of my life. It's one of the best things about my job.

I've been exposed to lots of different sectors. I've done work in corporate organisations, schools and universities. I've travelled up and down the country, meeting all sorts of people. A few stick out in my memory.

It was lovely visiting Kier Construction. Raising awareness of mental ill-health in the construction industry is vital, as there are very high rates of suicide in that sector, which made sharing my story with a group of (mainly male) construction workers especially important. I spoke honestly and openly about my eating disorder, admitting all those things about my brain that not long ago I would have found so embarrassing to admit.

I went into my talk with the expectation that no one would speak to me afterwards, assuming that it would be quite a "man-up" type culture. But it was absolutely brilliant – when I finished talking there were men of all ages waiting to talk, ask questions and share their experiences.

Some opportunities led to some incredibly meaningful moments for me, and for this reason I really enjoyed filming for *Nursing Times*. It gave me the opportunity to reunite with the lovely Mandy, one of the nurses in the hospital I stayed in who often went running with me. It was surreal catching up with her, to the point that I felt a serious mixture of nerves and excitement in the run-up to it. I hadn't seen Mandy since my discharge day ten and a half years ago. I wondered what she'd think when she saw me. I wondered how I'd feel about seeing someone who had seen me at some of my lowest points.

We talked openly about recovery, reflecting on my time at the unit and chatting about the things that Anorexia had made me do when I had been in the grips of it. For the interview we were asked to think about the role that Mandy had taken in supporting me in my exercise. And as I sat there, I realised the absolutely amazing care she had given me. Yes, there were points when I would get angry at her – mainly when she had wanted me to run slower! – but she was instrumental in my recovery and gave me long-lasting coping mechanisms, which have helped my recovery further. Often we take caregivers for granted, and I'm sure I did, but I know that the time, effort and relationship I had with Mandy has helped me get to where I am now.

In May 2018 I ended up going back to Michael Page, a company I had spent a year working in straight after I graduated. I did the talk alongside Jonny Benjamin MBE, a prominent mental health activist, and Neil Laybourn, the man who stopped him from jumping off a bridge. It was scary but exciting to share a platform with them. It made everything feel legitimate. I had really struggled during my time there – not with the work, but having to have a full-time job when I felt so uneasy about food. Some days I didn't know what to eat, in fear that maybe my workmates would judge my meals. The hours were long and hard, but only because they interfered with my exercise routine. I never talked to anyone about how I felt and I didn't tell anyone about my anorexia. I had been very closed off from them, and so it felt so strange to walk back through those doors, back to the place I wore a mask every morning, hiding my true feelings.

I didn't always know the final outcome of my talks, but I think the very act of sharing stories will always help people and give them some hope. I want everyone everywhere to know that recovery is possible, that Anorexia is a manipulative bitch and not worth being friends with.

CHAPTER 3

CREATING REAL CHANGE

As my work as a public speaker continued, I began to think more about how I could make long-term, strategic changes and how to take the conversation that little bit further. This was when I managed to secure my first platform in parliament in March 2018. I had just five minutes or so to present to the Labour Mental Health Group. I already had some ideas of what I wanted to see happen, so I was excited to have the chance to share my thoughts.

As I approached the stand, I looked and realised that I was slightly nervous. But I was also desperate to make change happen. I shared my story and then talked about the transition from children to adult services at eighteen and the lack of understanding around eating disorders when it comes to diagnosis. It was a terrifying but thrilling experience and I left wanting to be an MP!

What I did realise at this event was that I wanted to make real, long-term change. I loved what I did with my speaking engagements, but I wanted to take this further and do something tangible. I wanted to improve the whole system, so that everyone can access the care they need.

It was at this point that I decided the best way for me to do this would be to launch a campaign.

'So, what are you going to do about it?' I was asked this question a lot whenever I talked about being turned away from services for not being thin enough, which always resulted in others telling me about their similar experiences. The question always stuck with me. It bothered me an awful lot that despite NICE (National Institute for Health and Care Excellence) guidelines, there was still this complete injustice happening for so many people with eating disorders. People were turned away constantly for not meeting a really low BMI threshold, even though they were already ill.

So I had to do something. Anything. This is the funny thing about me – I am very good at taking work risks, but in my personal life I lack confidence to do that. Pretty much the whole campaign was planned in a pub using napkins and receipts, and after this I decided I was committed to tackling this head on.

As a result, my #DumpTheScales campaign launched in 2018.

#DumpTheScales had two main aims: firstly, to make sure the government realised the seriousness of eating disorders and that they enforced the national clinical guidance so that people weren't turned away from services for not being a low enough weight. Secondly, it was about giving others a voice and changing societal attitudes around eating disorders. For so long we think that people with eating disorders have to be stick thin and look like skeletons, but this is so far from the truth.

Admittedly, at first, I didn't think much would happen. I wanted it to, but I wasn't entirely sure how I would get very far with it. The petition launched on 6th July 2018, and I was expecting to get maybe ten or twenty signatures. But over the next few days, the momentum began to build. I did an event that weekend in Wantage, and on my way back the numbers suddenly began to increase at a fast rate. I couldn't quite believe it.

As the media coverage picked up, I realised I was going to need more planning and engagement work with the government. I was hearing even more stories of people who were struggling with this issue, people who were constantly being turned away for not having a ridiculously low BMI. It was saddening to realise the number of people who had experienced this – even I hadn't realised the true extent of the problem. The responses to the campaign flooded in daily and I struggled to keep up with them, but it also made me even more determined to fight.

At the end of November, I sat in parliament while my petition got debated, and I became overwhelmed with emotion. I had worked tirelessly to get it this far and I knew that while we had a long way to go, it was such a positive step in the right direction. The government was were now actually talking about eating disorders, and having my name mentioned in parliament concerning a project I was leading just felt amazing.

I contacted key ministers and began working with MPs such as Wera Hobhouse, Preet Kaur-Gill, Dr Rosena Khan, Caroline Nokes and Chris Evans, further championing our cause. It was a long process, but over time things began to pick up. By February 2019, the petition had hit 72,000 signatures. And there it sat for the next few months. I continued to work on it and meet with ministers, but I was slightly frustrated that it was slowing down. I needed the government to take it more seriously.

On 11th April 2019, we took the petition to Downing Street. It was a surreal, amazing experience to walk down Downing Street with journalists from the BBC and ITV present. Finally, I was delivering what I had worked on for so long.

The frustration came a few weeks later when I received their answer in the form of a letter. It was such a stock response. It focused far too much on children's services and on the NHS ten-year plan. It was upsetting because it felt like the government wasn't taking this issue seriously. The fact is, you can function for a long time with an eating disorder, but it isn't a way of life. It wasn't okay that the government weren't acting on this.

The petition was frustrating me at this point. Honestly, if it wasn't for those supporting me with it, I don't know whether I could have kept the momentum going as I did. It was my passion and my purpose to do this, but at times it still felt hard.

On Friday 28th June, I headed to the BBC studio to film with *BBC Sunday Politics*. I was to be interviewed alongside Jackie

Doyle-Price, Minister for Mental Health. I was worried about this interview. I tended to be okay with media, but for some reason this made me anxious. Thankfully I got though it all fine, and what followed over the next twenty-four hours was a huge increase in petition numbers. It reached 92,000! I was amazed. I was re-invigorated and inspired to work on this campaign once more. Here was another chance to make real change

Running a campaign has its highs and lows, but I absolutely love doing it. I have enjoyed it every step of the way. It's so rewarding to champion the rights of people with eating disorders and work to ensure that positive change happens. I have learnt a lot over the last year, and I have won two awards for my hard work in trying to change the system. I have learnt a lot not only about politics, but also about how long things take to change.

I always want things to happen quickly, so I do get frustrated with the pace. But you know what? We will get there. And I won't stop until we do.

CHAPTER 4

TIPS FOR DEALING WITH ANOREXIA

As a public speaker on mental health issues, particularly anorexia, I'm often asked to give tips and advice for fellow sufferers. So I thought I would offer some help to people for two of the hardest situations you'll face when in recovery from an eating disorder (ones that I think really hit a nerve for me): travelling and Christmas Day (or any other festive occasion that you might celebrate in your culture that typically involves a lot of food). Both are widely considered as fun, positive activities, but actually for people with anorexia or an eating disorder, they can be really stressful.

Travelling

In October 2017, I had a wobble about an upcoming trip. I was heading to Taiwan for a few weeks and had no idea what the food would be like, how much I'd be exercising, and what would affect my mood. The biggest thing playing on my mind was that the last time I'd gone on holiday for that long, I'd gone to Sri Lanka. And that had been the start of a tough year. That had been the year that Anorexia had tried to come back in to my life, the year I'd lost my grandma, the year I'd battled a relapse and suicidal thoughts. That was the year when I'd nearly ended everything, because I was struggling to cope and I thought people would be better off without the hassle of me relapsing. And so, this time around, I felt nervous that something else could go wrong again.

Generally, though, travelling really helps my recovery. It keeps me motivated and reminds me to keep moving forward, and it actually helped me start the recovery process in the first place. But travelling when in recovery isn't always easy; in fact it can, at times, be rather challenging, especially when making the right food choices becomes difficult. You don't always know when the next meal is and you don't know what it will be.

But you don't have to let that stop you exploring the world!

Here are my top tips for you:

1. If you're struggling, talk about it. Have people that you can check in with on a daily basis and tell them how you're finding it. This needs to be someone you trust, so that you can ask for reassurance about your worries and confirmation that you are having enough food.

2. Have an "easy" day if you need it. Sometimes on holiday I have a tuna day! This means I basically have meals and food I don't find challenging. It helps me enjoy the rest of the holiday and I don't feel guilty about it as it helps me stay well! So if you need to, gravitate towards the food that you already feel comfortable with, so that you can continue to enjoy your trip.

3. Don't get caught up in thinking about what you ate the previous day, and don't overthink the food! Remind yourself that you know it won't have an impact on others if they change their food for a week or two, so how is it any different for you?

4. Distract yourself if you are starting to let your mind drift to calories or the food. Get involved in an activity. Go sightseeing. Find something else, something fun, to occupy your mind until the thought passes.

5. Remind yourself that it doesn't matter if your portions are bigger than those at home. That's completely normal. It's nothing to be ashamed of. Life is too short to feel ashamed. Let's keep living!

Christmas (or festive occasions)

Christmas is hard. It comes with a lot of expectation and focus on food. For me, just getting through the day was amazing and a huge achievement in itself. But what I didn't realise was that the next day was going to be even harder. Waking up on Boxing Day, I felt the guilt set in. I felt *guilty* that I had actually had a really good day. I needed so badly to get some sense of normality back.

It is on days like these that Anorexia begins to creep back, slowly seducing you, sucking you back in, calling out for you in the dead of the night during those quiet moments. She knew just when to hit me. When I was half way round Wandsworth Common, running and feeling completely free, she hit me like a tonne of bricks.

'Hope, what the hell were you doing yesterday? Seriously, come on. You should *not* have enjoyed that day.'

They just kept on coming – these emotions, these feelings. That voice ridiculed me, came at me from all angles. I hated it. I had to fight it. I had to stay strong, summon all my energy and push myself further through it. I had to argue with Anorexia, loud and clear! I told her to back down and leave me alone. *Fight, fight, fight!* I shouted at myself. I wanted absolutely nothing to do with Anorexia anymore; I could live my life without her. The guilt fought back, but I fought on. Sometimes that's what we have to do: pull every bit of strength we have in order to move onwards and upwards. We may feel emotionally and physically exhausted, but it will be worth pulling through in the end.

It *is* possible to enjoy Christmas – and birthdays and other big get-togethers – and not go through this kind of torment. But it takes a bit of planning. Here's some advice for both sufferers of anorexia and their loved ones. Hopefully they will help you get through it and have a good time:

1. **Have set times for the mealtimes**. A huge anxiety for me around Christmas is the fact that lunch, for some reason, needs to be served in the middle of the afternoon, and regardless of the time they promise to serve it, it is often late. It means that I feel anxious about the food, then I get all psyched up, and then I'm let

down. Asking if people can stick to set serving times can be a real game changer for people with eating disorders, and normally isn't an issue for other people.

2. Ask if you can see the menu beforehand. Knowing what is on offer is essential for many. I used to like to know this so that I could plan for meals and know whether to have my morning snack or not. I recommend this for all the meals around the festive day. My mum and I did just this at Christmas, and I also cooked the Christmas lunch.

3. Get help with portion sizes. Do I have three or four roast potatoes? What should I have? Portion size is an absolute minefield when you are in recovery, and at Christmas this becomes even harder (especially for me – I grew up with two brothers who could eat more than ten roast potatoes in one sitting). If you're someone who is supporting a person with anorexia, offer them advice on portion size, but don't be forceful if they think they have had enough, as you need to be mindful to not lose their trust. (One thing that my mum does when we go for buffets is to suggest that I just have a similar portion to her, which always helps.)

4. If you are supporting a loved one with anorexia, offer them a quick twenty minute walk to vent. Getting out on Christmas Day is important for everyone (I think!) but for people with eating disorders, having that chance to stretch their legs and vent in a safe place if they have found it tough is good. I always recommend offering this, away from any food, as it will hopefully allow the person breathing space and allow them to be more comfortable. On Christmas Day this year I went for a quick night-time stroll on my own, and it was lovely. It gave me some space and some alone time. I need my space, and it is essential that I find a way to manage this in a healthy way.

5. Remember, you don't always have to know the answers. That's why surrounding yourself with people who know how hard it is is so important, if you are lucky enough to have people in your life who you can trust. Eating disorders are really complicated and are unique to each individual, but the important thing is that you are with someone who will be there for you. For supporters of people with anorexia, be patient, even when that feels hard. And remember that the eating disorder may make that individual do something nasty that they wouldn't normally do. Just being there is essential – for me, knowing that I have my family rooting for me to keep going and get through Christmas Day is what I need.

6. Tell the person with an eating disorder that you know how hard it is, and that it is okay if they're not feeling okay. Make a conscious effort to say this on the morning of the big day. Something that I really struggled with in my recovery was beginning to eat and being a healthy weight, but still not feeling 100% okay about it all. I used to worry that by eating and enjoying food, people would think I was completely better. If you act on only one of my suggestions this Christmas or festive period, please do this one! Remind the person you are supporting that festivities and celebrations are hard, and that you get that. Remind them you want to support them and want to help. Tell them that you won't assume they're okay if they eat and enjoy the food. This always helped take away my guilt about food.

7. Remember that it is only one day, and eat meals you are more comfortable with before or after the main event. This may seem like a simple one, but for people with eating disorders, Christmas Day (or other festive days) can feel like a monster you have to fight and beat. It feels like getting through the day is unachievable, like it will never end. I used to make sure I had meals I felt comfortable with each side of Christmas Day. This allowed me to feel more in control. I learnt that I didn't have to eat everything in sight, and that once I had made it through this day, I would feel better about what I was eating.

8. Be aware of those around you. Around Christmas time and New Year, conversations completely evolve around food, calories, and dieting. The reality is, it is such a nightmare for everyone! But for people with eating disorders or people in recovery there is that nagging feeling that maybe you should give up fighting and lose that weight.

From the age of twelve, all of my new year resolutions revolved around diets, avoiding snacking, and exercise. Every year, that is, until I turned seventeen, my heart nearly stopped and I was admitted in to a mental health hospital, where I spent the next year of my life battling to get well.

So this January, please be aware of those around you and think before you start loudly discussing how much weight you are going to lose or the number of calories you are going to cut. Yes, it may seem annoying to have to stop these conversations, but it can seriously trigger other people and cause them huge anxiety.

CHAPTER 5

CHALLENGING MY RECOVERY

When you wake up in the morning and look in the mirror, what is the first thing you think about? Are you happy with what you see? Do you look at yourself and feel disgusted? How do you feel as the day progresses – do you feel better or worse about your appearance? If you hate what you see so much, do you give up on the day, write it off and go back to bed?

I have days when I look in the mirror and feel okay, while on other days I try on my entire wardrobe before heading out to work, feeling huge. It's during these times that I remind myself that I've come a long way. But the road to recovery has its setbacks. It is anything but smooth.

In May 2018, I realised that once again my life had become dictated by food. I wasn't great at branching out anymore and I had lost all confidence in listening to my body. It was hard not to go back to what had been an easy routine before and I think sometimes I just couldn't be bothered to be risky in my meal choices. I had this realisation that I was eating the same meals every week and drinking the same amount of alcohol. My life was still massively controlled by anorexia. I hated that part of my mind, but I didn't really know what to do about it. *Perhaps I will always be like this, I thought to myself. Perhaps I'll always be stuck in this rut, just living as a functioning anorexic.*

But the fact was, I didn't want to be like this. I knew I needed to discipline myself and challenge my recovery. I wanted to branch out and have food I actually *wanted*. It wasn't about having absolutely terrifying meals every day, but just having food I enjoyed. I wanted to go out, not always knowing where I was going to eat and not knowing what would be cooked for me. It was about listening to my body and eating what I wanted to eat, not what that part of my brain might be telling me to.

As I committed to this, I became quite scared. What if I lost all control? Would everyone think I was totally okay now if they saw me eating a pizza? What if I put on weight? What if the anorexia just disappeared? Surely that would be a good thing if it did, but then would I feel things again. I'd have no defences against my emotions.

But I told myself that despite these fears, I was going to push myself every day to do this. And I knew that the only way I could do it properly was to tell the people around me, so I had people that I was accountable to.

And so it began, the long drag of challenging myself. Below are some snippets of my tweets that helped me keep track of my journey.

17th May 2018

Last Sunday I wrote myself a list of challenges. I have become far too comfy living in recovery from anorexia and I have stopped pushing myself. This often means that when I go for dinner, I pick restaurants that I find easy or pick stuff off the menu that I may not really want, but is manageable.

Tonight I thought, *fuck it, I am going to risk it! I am going to eat a real beef burger!* I hadn't had one of these since before I became unwell (aged thirteen). But I did it! I'm not entirely sure how I feel about it and in the back of my brain I'm slightly worried, but I don't care! Challenging anorexia is bringing me one step closer to getting that voice out of my life completely! And I know I am stronger than all those thoughts. I am 100% stronger than Anorexia, that manipulative bitch who ruins lives!

19th July 2018

Challenging myself tonight at Mercato Metropolitano in order to beat that relentless anorexic voice! I find market food quite stressful and anorexia sometimes tries to make me pick the "healthiest" or "low-calorie" option, mainly so Anorexia shuts up and doesn't make me feel guilty ... But tonight, I picked something I actually wanted! And while I feel slightly guilty for doing that, I know I can beat that voice because listening to it does NOTHING!

1st August 2018

Challenging my brain and focusing on my recovery food after a cycle today! I won't let Anorexia dictate what I can and can't eat anymore! Food is fuel, and it should not be about the calories!

15th November 2018

Yesterday I had quite a tough day, with the anorexic voice causing real havoc in my brain! I don't get days like this much anymore, but when I do, I get so frustrated with myself, partly because of how the voice makes me feel – like a fat, insecure failure – but also because I feel slightly hypocritical.

So last night, after speaking to the Yes Tribe, I thought, *F*** you, Anorexia!* I am going to go out for a spontaneous meal and have something I don't normally eat!

For those of you who know me, you will know I struggle with rice, and definitely totally non-portion-controlled rice! But I did it! I stuck two fingers up to Anorexia and I am still standing today! And I actually feel good today! Some days in recovery that voice will shout louder and louder, but stick with the fight, because I guarantee it will get easier and is totally worth it!

8th April 2019

Challenge one of the weekend was trying pork scratchings! Before I got unwell, I used to love crackling! And despite only having a couple from the packet I am pleased I challenged myself.

Challenge two was chicken, leek and bacon pie, and although I feel a bit guilty saying this, I really enjoyed it. Pushing boundaries in recovery is hard at times, but it is so worth doing! Sometimes for me, the hardest part is waking up the next morning. This happened when I had the pie. I panicked, lying there in bed, my hand running over my tummy. Was I feeling it right? Was it really a bit bigger? When this happens, I have to remind myself what Anorexia does. She really is a lying bitch at times!

Challenges are a key part of my recovery, and the more I do them, the better things are. Yes, they are hard, and at times I absolutely hate doing them, but they are crucial for me. This is the way I see it: if I don't constantly push my recovery, then I will feel the need to restrict again. Anorexia makes me look more inwardly. Over time, it might cause me to not put spread on my toast, or cut out sauces, or completely cut out certain food groups. That is the scary thing with anorexia – it creeps in at times, slowly sucking you back in.

I knew I didn't want that to ever happen again, so I needed to be proactive and battle it. I do really believe that there is something in this for all of us. In recovery, we have to push the boundaries of what the anorexia is telling us, challenging ourselves so that we can actually start living fully. There is a huge difference between thriving and surviving, and for so long I simply survived. Maybe at times I still do, but the fact is now I am pushing forward and doing my best to thrive.

I don't see myself as a functioning anorexic, but I see myself as someone in recovery. For me, the difference is that functioning anorexics let Anorexia control their lives, but actively pushing back is what puts people in recovery. Recovery is accepting that some days I will find it hard, and that that is okay. It's fine to have difficult feelings, but it's what you do with them that makes a difference.

I didn't just challenge myself with food. Exercise had always been a massive part of my illness. At my worst, I had it in my head that I had to exercise whenever I ate in order to be thin. And so when I was in hospital, I had to completely reteach myself what normal exercise was.

It has been a long journey, but now I exercise in a healthy way, vary up my workouts, have rest days and eat enough to fuel myself. And that's why, again in 2018, I felt healthy enough to take on JOGLE – a charity bike ride from John O'Groats to Land's End – on behalf of the Shaw Mind Foundation.

I am not entirely sure why I agreed to do it, to be honest, but it felt like an amazing idea. I figured that, since I was a long-distance runner, it surely wouldn't be that hard to become good at cycling. I began my training over the summer, heading to Richmond Park and doing lap after lap before work. I loved the challenge, but I knew deep down I had to be really careful not to damage myself or my recovery.

I needed a huge amount of guidance on food and my training plan. Accepting that help was crucial, and I knew that – while admittedly it was slightly annoying having people checking in with me – it would also help keep Anorexia at bay and make things feel less difficult in my head.

One of the hardest things I have had to get my head round with all my cycling training is making sure I'm fuelling myself enough. But I hated failing, and I knew that if I let my doubts around food creep in when I was trying to fuel myself sufficiently, Anorexia would get the better of me. And that would be a guaranteed failure.

The trip started positively. I had a bit of a hiccup on 25th September, my third day in, when the wind and rain began and I ended up falling off my bike on an A-road. It was scary, but the good news is that I can now put on a bike chain very easily! The two weeks that followed merged in to this sea of tired legs, pub dinners, nut bars and *so much water*. The end was getting closer, but still at times it felt so far off. The second week was particularly tough, and by the time I had gone through Bristol I was struggling to keep going. Physically I was exhausted, but mentally I needed to find a way to be strong.

I knew I did not want to fail.

As I approached the final day of JOGLE, I wasn't sure I would make it. It was all beginning to feel too hard and I wasn't quite sure what to do about it. I cried a lot, both hating what I was doing and trying to love it at the same time. I had to constantly remind myself why I was doing it – for mental health. To raise money and awareness. I couldn't give up now.

Crossing that finish line was surreal. I finished at 11.30 am after a 5 am start. The rain and wind were battering me down and I could barely hear myself think as I arrived at the finish line. But I had done it! I had successfully cycled the length of the UK.

What I didn't realise was how much of an impact it would have on me when the bike ride finished. I got back to London and weighed myself. I wanted to make sure that I was in a good place physically.

My weight hadn't budged at all.

While this was a really good thing, Anorexia immediately piped up in my head.

'If anyone else had done this, they would have lost so much weight. You will lose control now if you don't keep cycling this much every day.'

I guess this really was a challenge to my recovery. I could feel myself slipping again, slowly but surely, and I knew I had to get back into my work and routine. I needed to claw back some control in order to stay well. Luckily, I had predicted a bit of a comedown after JOGLE (I think this happens quite often to lots of people after big sporting events or times of business) and so the week afterwards was extremely full on. It helped me get through, but it masked my feelings. I didn't embrace the fact that I was struggling again with food and exercise, and instead I began to let the anorexia seep back in.

I felt frustrated, but I also knew that this time I could be stronger than this. And I *wanted* to be. I wanted to be able to hold on to all my strength and positivity and push myself in the right direction. And so I cut myself some slack. I went back to my amazing personal trainer, Lyndsey, who knows a lot about my back history, and managed to get well before it all slipped away again.

The takeaway from all of this is that throughout recovery, there will be these moments where things get harder. There'll be times when you see yourself at a crossroads and you have to make a decision. And that's okay.

Keep fighting back. Keep telling Anorexia she won't win.

CHAPTER 6

REALISATIONS

For the last two and a half years – in the time since I started sharing my personal story of recovery – I have had real highs and real lows. Don't get me wrong, I love doing what I do, and it is a huge part of my life now. I wouldn't change it for anything. But it does essentially mean I'm reliving my trauma on a regular basis. And it doesn't make me immune to feeling like shit, to having to deal with general aching and dullness at times. I am also very empathetic, and that can be tough at times, especially since I want to help everyone and always put others ahead of myself. Up until July 2019, I was actually convinced that my needs didn't matter as much as others, and as long as everyone else was happy, that was okay.

When I start to feel unhappy, I tend to go into this full-on practical mode. I find as soon as I feel unhappy or uncomfortable, it makes my guard go right back up. I basically do what I tell everyone else not to do to me, and try to fix myself. It is frustrating in and of itself, but over the last few months, focusing on my job has caused me to lose so much of what I love and want from life.

I always said I wouldn't be one of those people who loses themselves to work, but for some reason I haven't been able to help it. This job is my passion, but I think more recently it has just become an escape from dealing with life. I am strong and I am in a much better place than I have ever been since my relapse, but still have to be mindful of what's really going on in my head.

In January 2019, my work began to pick up and move even faster. In the first year of working for myself, I was doing lots of unpaid work and not really actually getting that much paid work. But I began my second year with weeks and weeks of talks booked up. The positive was that I was not quite as stressed about money, but it also meant that the more I worked, the more distant I became. I became so focused on my passion for changing the world that I wasn't thinking about the key things in my life that mattered.

I threw myself into everything so that I didn't have to deal with actually how I was feeling. I would head off and do a talk and feel amazing, getting the highs and lows that so many people get from "performing", but what I had not yet managed to do was deal with my emotions. And so, throughout the start of 2019, I began to lose things important things in my life that meant so much to me. They were slipping away.

The frustrating thing was, I was in this false sense of illusion. I continuously told myself that things would be okay when life quietened down, that I could prioritise better then. But it didn't happen that way. I justified evening work by squeezing in an hour here and there with people, and it all added up.

My work/life balance was a mess, but for some reason I wasn't doing anything about it. I would spend every opportunity I had working or managing my social media. I went on Sky News to talk about how people are obsessed with their phones, when really, I am one of those people. I kept justifying my actions and behaviours by claiming that I needed to have my phone all the time, that I had to be ready for media enquiries, that I had to be around in case someone needed me (I get a lot of messages from people who are struggling). But it was getting to the point when I was on my phone at all hours, and I would even check my messages and emails in the middle of the night when I got up to go for a wee. Whenever I got on the train or I was waiting for something to happen, I would just get sucked back into work instead of being in the moment. I was that girl that just talked about work all the time.

It came to a climax in May 2019. It was a funny month, one with lots of plans and high expectations. But none really came together. Instead I felt unsettled and full of unease. I decided I needed a therapist and that was okay, so I set off for my first session. She told me in the first session that I didn't deal with my emotions in a healthy way (no brainer!). I knew that, but I didn't know how to process them correctly. So, instead of going back to work it out, I convinced myself that £100 was far too much for a therapist and I would rather spend money on new trainers, getting my hair done, or my nails ... because surely that would help just as much?

Mental Health Awareness Week came, and I had four talks booked per day. And to think that at one time I was worried about getting nothing! I was as booked up as I could be, but I was excited about it. I went into the week feeling so positive about everything, and I survived it, despite a few hiccups.

But the week after that, my life began to feel like it was falling apart. I ended up standing on a train, travelling between work appointments, crying my eyes out with my face shoved up against the glass.

Why had I let myself get so out of control? Why had I once again become one of those people who wears a mask every day to pretend like life is okay? Why had I let my relationships slip? Yes, I wanted to save the world, and I am so unbelievably passionate about mental health. But at the same time things were becoming dangerous. Life was uncomfortable because my emotions were triggered once again, so instead of managing it, I focused on others and dismissed myself.

I had got so used to ignoring the warning signs, investing so much time in others and focusing far too much on my campaign. I really loved my job and I knew that I could do it, but I had to be in the right frame of mind and I needed to make sure I didn't burn out. I had focused more on fixing others than myself. As a result, I needed to get the rest of my life back on track. I knew my mind and I knew the warning signs and I talked about the power of talking. But for some reason, while I alluded to feeling stressed from time to time, I wasn't able to really be that honest about myself. Sometimes the hardest thing is admitting to yourself and those around you that you aren't okay. Being in my line of work, I also feel slightly paranoid about admitting things. I worried about the impact it would have on people booking me in to speak, or whether schools would think I couldn't possibly come in now. That's the thing – I believe there is stigma within the mental health community, and I think I felt it. I was afraid of reaching out, because I knew that from the outside, I looked like I was doing just fine. People always told me how strong I was – and yes, I am – but I was still breaking.

It all came to a head on Monday 8th July. I headed into town early to meet my friend for coffee. I was pleased I was out of the house, as I wasn't doing that well when I was on my own (another warning sign!). I walked down the road towards the café, Rapha, and on seeing him I burst into tears. I don't know what came over me. I was shaking, trying so hard to swallow back my tears. I wasn't okay.

We sat for hours in the café chatting, processing, venting. And it set me up for the day. The rest of the day was okay and I was back to conning myself that maybe everything was okay again. Maybe I was actually okay.

On Tuesday 9th July I woke up early, heading to the gym before a meeting in town. I felt completely empty, afraid and so lonely. My brain felt cold and broken and I was feeling so much pain I didn't know what to think or do. And yet I still pulled myself together, showered, put on my make-up and donned a nice dress (because surely if I looked presentable, then it would be okay). I sent a few messages about Dump the Scales, coming up with new ideas and plans as a good distraction. I arrived at my meeting acting bubbly, cheery and in full swing.

I was touring a specialist eating disorder clinic in Central London. I looked longingly at the "sitting room" where the clients were, wishing I was just sitting in there, getting some support. Then we headed up to the top floor to meet with the CEO; he was talking and I was only half-listening (another warning sign). I wasn't engaged and I didn't know what was wrong with me; I had to keep pushing myself to listen and it was taking every bit of energy I had. The meeting finished and I had surprised myself by managing to get through it.

I headed back to Oxford Street, focusing on my emails and social media along the way. I got to the station and headed for the Victoria line. I was going to another meeting at Kings Cross, so I was relieved to get a seat on the Tube.

It was then that the emotion hit me.

I tried so hard to swallow my tears, but I couldn't do it. They kept coming, whirling in my eyes and trickling down my face. The lady opposite me moved to sit next to me and put her arm round me (surely crying on the Tube is the biggest warning sign ever). I wasn't feeling suicidal or even thinking about ending my life. I just wasn't okay. My problem wasn't with food this time, but my mood.

I had ten minutes before I had to make a call, and then had a meeting in Leon at midday. I had to do this. I needed help and I had to start practising what I preached. I knew I had to do something or this was going to escalate.

I have these moments in my life when I realise that something isn't right. We all probably do. Sometimes I act on them and sometimes I don't. The plan was quite straightforward; there was nothing super magical about it. I crafted a message to a few people close to me. The message was simple: 'I am not okay and I think I need some help. Thank you for being so patient with me, and I am sorry.'

As I pressed send, I was worried about what people would say, whether people would think I was weak. All that stigma still surrounds mental health, despite all the work I'd been doing.

I had some quick, instant replies, which was amazing. Most of them said well done, telling me it was okay, and asking me what the plan was. Well, this was step one: telling those closest to me, getting reassurance and bringing back together my army of people to help me fight.

Step two was acting on it, which is just as hard. I decided I didn't want everyone to know about this just yet, so I contacted someone at my local hospital who I trusted, and asked if they could help with therapy. I also booked a GP appointment. Having spent a lot of my life questioning what had caused my anorexia in the first place, I felt the need to do this now. I wanted to get to the bottom of it, so I knew what I needed – four to six weeks of intensive therapy to help me get back on track.

Before this point, I'd never been able to get my brain fully and honestly engaged in therapy. I'd done lots of it, but I still found the emotional aspect really challenging. However, I knew this time it would be different.

I wanted to return to the "real" me quickly, but I had to understand that these things take time. And you know what? That is totally okay, for me and for you.

Not long afterwards, I went on a last-minute trip to Majorca with a friend. I used to do stuff like this all the time; I was once totally spontaneous. But it had stopped over the last year. During this trip I was the most relaxed I had been in ages, and I guess that was helped along by my two weeks of intensive therapy, admitting that I was not okay, and spending time with a wonderful person, Tatjana, who exudes positivity.

We sat for hours chatting (and tanning ... well, burning!) on the beach, and as we did so, I came to some realisations about what had caused my recent distress and low mood:

1. I had become a work-a-holic. I'd let so much slide in the last year, such as friendships, quality time with my partner, and so much more. I love my job, so that was a factor in my overworking, but I also used work to ignore my emotions while working, and that was far less positive.

2. I had tried to please too many people. I always wanted others to be happy, and would rather put others ahead of my own happiness. But this sometimes meant that my priorities got all skewed. One weekend, there had been a problem with my family, and so I headed home. This would have been fine normally, but I hadn't seen my partner properly for quality time. He felt shelved by all this, but I didn't know what to do or how to juggle things. And again, instead of tackling the issue, I worked harder still. It was as if I had to prioritise work to proof myself ... or maybe I was self-destructing a bit! I was annoyed that I had lost the real Hope, and in the process, I was losing people close to me. And I'd been in so much denial about it.

3. I was always letting people get to me. There are a certain few people who I'd really struggled with over the last few years. I worried a lot about them, spending a lot of time reading into their behaviours, questioning my own worth when I was around them. Just after Christmas, I'd gone through a period where I had to have some really difficult conversations with a few people. I went into each discussion feeling nervous, but trying to be positive. Sometimes the discussions went well, but I'd still read into things the other person said, convincing myself I wasn't good enough or capable of dealing with things. These behaviours began to escalate, to the point that I started hating life. In fact, I had been in this negative spiral for quite a long time. I was fine on the surface, especially when I was working with people, but I'd find myself right back in that black hole whenever I was alone. It was frustrating for me, but instead of tackling the issue, I burrowed it deeper.

4. I always focused on fixing others rather than embracing my feelings. This seems to be a recurring theme here!

5. I'd reported my sexual abuse back in September, without thinking about how I'd deal with the emotional impact. It was a massive thing for me to do, and it was so hard releasing something out into the world that I'd boxed up for so long. I thought I was

strong enough to go through it without any professional support at the time, but then I'd started experiencing flashbacks. Surely this should have been a warning sign, but no! Instead I let it get the better of me, building up my guard to protect myself. And again, all this did was hurt those closest to me. The scary thing with sexual abuse is the hold it has over for you for so long; it can result in unconscious behaviours towards those around you. The other thing is that you have to jump through so many obstacles to report a case. In my situation, it ended up being his word against mine, so they dropped the case. This rocked me like nothing had ever done before, and it had that effect on me throughout the entire investigation.

6. I'd changed, and not in a way that I liked. I had stopped living life the way I used to, as a fun, carefree girl. Instead, I always found myself so caught up with things. I thought maybe part of this was because I was approaching my thirties, but it went deeper than that. As a result, I had been left with so much anger and resentment, mostly towards myself. I'd started to judge myself, panicking when I had to see certain people. During some events I'd panic for hours beforehand and get into a right state, knowing that a certain woman would be there. It was strange and so unlike me. Yes, I had my insecurities, but they'd never made me act this way before. I began to resent certain situations too, and at times for no real reason. Yes, I could function like this for a long time. But eventually there had to come a time for me to challenge it. I had to accept that I had lost myself along the way, and going away with Tatjana had helped me do this.

Some people might beat themselves up for taking so long to get help, thinking of all the things they've missed out on. And yes, I was annoyed at myself for taking so long to reach out for support, but what's the point in mulling it over? I'd messed up in so many ways, but actually this could be the start of something new, something that would make me stronger. The right people would wait for me to come out the other side.

I also wanted to become more positive. I'd read the memes online, but they weren't really working, so I needed to be more hands on and focused! Therapy was amazing and a real game changer, but I needed to help myself in other ways too. So I followed Tatjana's brilliant advice, and it's already helped me a lot:

1. **Ask people for five things they love about you.** This sounds a bit bizarre, and it was a tough one for me. I felt a bit embarrassed that it was egocentric, but Tatjana assured me it wasn't. In fact, it made me feel great.

2. **Say yes more!** From holidays, to meals out, to last-minute drinks, just say yes. The old me would have done this, and I needed to get my love of life back.

3. **Have a feel-good folder on your phone**, which includes a list of things you love, positive affirmations, fun memories and positive feedback.

4. **Delete the things that make you feel rubbish**, whether it's music or certain people's numbers. Delete them and it will help!

5. **Think about who is around you.** What do they give you? We all have friends who we see because we have to, friends we struggle with. It's okay to leave them behind if it makes you feel better.

I am only into week four of all of this, but I'm actually already feeling stronger. I'm now able to turn my mood around within twenty minutes and I am now talking more! Amazingly, friends, family and the people I work with are already commenting on *me*. Not on my weight or my work or on my campaigning, but *me*. 'The old you is coming back,' they say, and that's what keeps me motivated!

Recovery has ups and downs and that is totally okay, but what really counts is how you press forward after a difficult time. One of the best things at the moment for me is my drive and determination to actually tackle this. I don't want this to be a sticking plaster; I don't want to leave a door slightly ajar in my brain for the anorexia and self-doubt to creep back in. I want to sort this out.

I know that it is going to be hard work getting back on track and feeling back to my old self completely again, but I also know it is totally worth doing. I am prepared for the battle to be back on. And I am prepared to beat it for once and for all. I don't want that gold medal for not eating; I want it for accomplishing this! And I know I will be stronger for it.

CHAPTER 7

ONWARDS

My story might seem like it's had lots of bumps along the way, but that's just life. Sharing all these issues I've had after the book came out is challenging; admitting it wasn't happily ever after is hard. But it's a fact of recovery, and that's something we all have to deal with. Yes, it can be frustrating at times, but the more you stick to positive plans, the easier it gets.

Besides, my journey is nowhere near finished yet. Over the last few weeks and years I have learnt so much about myself and about the people around me. I now know what really matters to me. Yes, it's taken me losing things to realise it, but that's okay. And for some people it will be too late, but again that's out of my control and I have to find a way to accept that.

There is so much more I hope to do with my life, from ending injustices for those with eating disorders and empowering others to speak out, to having my own family, helping solve the refugee crisis and seeing more of the world. It is these things that keep me pushing forward every day.

On a smaller level, I'm going to go back to those food challenges and actually do them every single day, celebrating them when I'm successful. I'm going to go back to finding a positive in every day and writing it down. I will spend time with friends who I haven't seen for ages, and, importantly, I will create some boundaries with work. I am going be okay with the fact that some days are quieter. It's time to start looking after my own wellbeing, too, and therapy is a huge part of that. I'm committed to cracking this once and for all. I've learnt a lot about my emotions already, and I appreciate that at the time of writing, my work here isn't completely done. But I now know what I need to do.

It's fine to be a work in progress, but that doesn't mean you should stop living your life, telling your story and changing things for the better. Don't let rock bottom terrify you. Anorexia is not worth listening to. I hid behind those false lies and false value for so long, and it doesn't work. Talking and feeling can be very hard, but it's so much better for you in the long run. It really will be okay.

If you find yourself relapsing after recovery, that doesn't make you a failure. You think people will judge you, that they'll think less of you, but they won't.

Admitting you are struggling after a relapse is powerful. It's also the start of a long road ahead of you, but it's helpful to remember that you're not starting from the beginning. This isn't square one. You can take what you already know and empower yourself with it.

So many of us go through these ups and downs. In fact, we all do. We all struggle from time to time to feel okay with life, the world, everything. What is important to remember is that when life just feels like it's spiralling out of control, you just need to take each day at a time. Learn to love yourself and talk. Come up with a plan of action. Small steps can be difficult, but they can also be life-changing in and of themselves, so I hope you can find inspiration in the small things I've discovered keep me motivated and feeling positive.

Stand up, and face the world, and fight. And remember – if you fall, you *can* and *will* come back stronger.

ACKNOWLEDGEMENTS

Thank you to Kate, James, Samuel and Mollie – the four of the famous five who are there with directness, support and unconditional love.

There are so many other people that I could think of to thank, those close to me who stood by me through thick and thin, and those who made me realise over the last year that I really needed help and didn't give up on me when I finally accepted it. You were there when I cried, you stayed when my guard was up, you were on the end of the phone, you gave me strength when I wanted to give up and you took my hand to pull me through. You kept me alive and fighting. Thank you for not giving up.

I also want to thank all those who supported my campaign, who put in time and effort to help it get to where it is. Thank you to my supporters and those in government who have helped me to increase my confidence and who believed in me and my campaign enough to push it higher up the agenda.

I would also like to thank Stephanie Cox for helping me bring my book to life. Not only has Steph been an amazing educator, but she has also been an amazing support emotionally.

TriggerHub.org is one of the most elite and scientifically proven forms of mental health intervention

Trigger Publishing is the leading independent mental health and wellbeing publisher in the UK and US. Clinical and scientific research conducted by assistant professor Dr Kristin Kosyluk and her highly acclaimed team in the Department of Mental Health Law & Policy at the University of South Florida (USF), as well as complementary research by her peers across the US, has independently verified the power of lived experience as a core component in achieving mental health prosperity. Specifically, the lived experiences contained within our bibliotherapeutic books are intrinsic elements in reducing stigma, making those with poor mental health feel less alone, providing the privacy they need to heal, ensuring they know the essential steps to kick-start their own journeys to recovery, and providing hope and inspiration when they need it most.

Delivered through TriggerHub, our unique online portal and accompanying smartphone app, we make our library of bibliotherapeutic titles and other vital resources accessible to individuals and organizations anywhere, at any time and with complete privacy, a crucial element of recovery. As such, TriggerHub is the primary recommendation across the UK and US for the delivery of lived experiences.

At Trigger Publishing and TriggerHub, we proudly lead the way in making the unseen become seen. We are dedicated to humanizing mental health, breaking stigma and challenging outdated societal values to create real action and impact. Find out more about our world-leading work with lived experience and bibliotherapy via triggerhub.org, or by joining us on:

🐦 @triggerhub_

ⓕ @triggerhub.org

▣ @triggerhub_

Printed in the USA
CPSIA information can be obtained
at www.ICGtesting.com
JSHW031713140824
68134JS00038B/3675